Interrupted Lives

Interrupted Lives

A History of Tuberculosis in Minnesota and Glen Lake Sanatorium

Mary Krugerud

NORTH STAR PRESS OF ST. CLOUD, INC.
St. Cloud, Minnesota

ISBN: 978-1-68201-065-5 (paper)
ISBN: 978-1-68201-082-2 (ebook)

First edition: September 2017

Printed in the United States of America.

Published by
North Star Press
19485 Estes Road
Clearwater, Minnesota 55320
www.northstarpress.com

Dedication

To:

~All former patients and employees of Glen Lake Sanatorium and Oak Terrace Nursing home, especially those who shared their memories and photos.

~Norma Anderson, who planted the seed for this book with her collection of interviews, *San Memories*.

~Colleen Spadaccini and Steve Perkins, fellow collaborators on the Glen Lake and Oak Terrace 75th anniversary documentary.

~Staff members at the Hopkins Historical Society, Hennepin History Museum, Minnetonka Historical Society, and the Minnesota History Center's Gale Library for assistance with this project.

~My family, because my interest in tuberculosis sanatoriums baffles them, and they support my efforts anyway.

TABLE OF CONTENTS

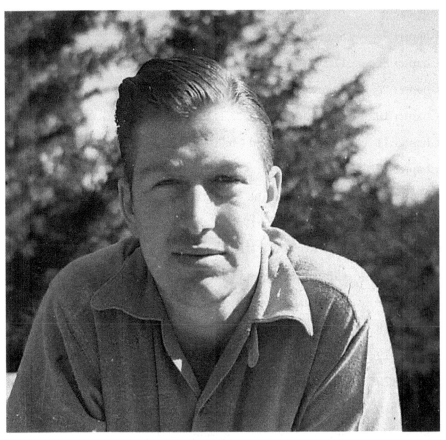

A young Frederick Manfred. (From the University of Minnesota Anderson Libary archives; used with the permission of the Manfred Literary Committee)

Introduction

March 1940. Feike Feikema, an unemployed journalist, is admitted to Glen Lake Sanatorium for treatment of tuberculosis. His bed is in the corner of a room he will share with three other men. An orderly tells Feikema that the previous occupant of that bed, a Finn named Toivo, was there sixteen years before he went home, cured. Feikema thinks, Holy smokes, sixteen years . . . Do I have to stay here that long? *Fifty years later, when he was a successful author known as Frederick Manfred, he recalled that he was too sick at the time to regard it with much alarm. "If you are vital and alive,"* he said, *"of course, then you think that is terrible. But when you're down to almost the last dregs of your life, you don't have any sense that it's terrible. You're just happy that for the moment you're feeding well and you're sleeping in a warm bed. So you don't think about that."*[1]

T HE SANATORIUM ERA, lasting approximately 100 years, played an import-ant role the control of tuberculosis in the United States. At the height of the era, more than 700 of the institutions existed in the United States, and their physicians and employees shared knowledge via organizations and conferences. Administrators worked closely with local anti-tuberculosis as-sociations on education campaigns. Doctors collaborated on milk pasteuri-zation legislation that made tuberculosis a preventable disease before it was curable. Non-medical staff at sanatoriums developed or influenced many now-common practices in the areas of educational, occupational and voca-tional therapies. Patients from several sanatoriums played a vital part in the search for a cure by volunteering to participate in drug trials.

Several books have reported on the medical history of tuberculosis and the social experience of illness. Many have focused on the first half of the sanatorium era, with its relentless monotony of bed rest and the absurdity of sleeping outside year-round. The total sanatorium experience from the patients' perspective is sparsely documented, however. The stigma of poverty or uncleanliness that accompanied tuberculosis meant that few who experienced a sanatorium were willing to talk about it. In addition, little of the existing literature informs us about children in tuberculosis sanatoriums.

In 1949, the Minnesota Public Health Association sponsored the publication of *Invited and Conquered: a Historical Sketch of Tuberculosis in Minnesota*. The author, J. Arthur Myers, M.D., detailed the history of tuberculosis in Minnesota from 1659 to 1949. Chapter Sixteen profiled sanatoriums operating at the time of publication, but the book's main focus was on the medical community involved in the state's fight against tuberculosis. Myers's assistant in gathering early background material was Theodore Streukens, a medical student who had been a patient at Glen Lake Sanatorium as a teenager. Tragically, Streukens's tuberculosis reactivated. He was re-admitted to the sanatorium, where he died in 1940.

More than 15,000 people sought a cure at Glen Lake Sanatorium in Hennepin County, Minnesota. The sanatorium is well-documented in the Minnesota Historical Society's archives. This wealth of information reveals a treatment regimen far more complex than just fresh air, rest, and sunshine. This book, based primarily on that collection, explores every facet of care and treatment at Glen Lake Sanatorium, including the children's preventorium and summer camp. In particular, it tells the story of one physician, Ernest S. Mariette, who was dedicated to creating what he called "the contented patient."

1

The White Plague in Minnesota

GLEN LAKE WAS PART OF A SYSTEM of sanatoriums authorized by the legislature to fight a contagious disease that, at the time, was the leading cause of death in the world. The sanatorium opened on January 4, 1916, to serve residents of Hennepin County, Minnesota, who had tuberculosis. A snowstorm on that day—described as a howling, icy gale—did not prevent a horse-drawn sleigh from transporting a buffalo-robed man twelve miles from St. Louis Park to the sanatorium.[1]

Dr. Herbert O. Collins, superintendent, extended the official greeting to Andrew Gibson, age forty-three. Gertrude Moore, resident nurse in charge, was among the greeters, along with Dr. Walter Marcley, a respected expert on tuberculosis. He had served as a surgeon for the U.S. Army during World War I and in various capacities with several hospitals and the Minnesota Department of Health. Dr. Ernest S. Mariette and twelve licensed nurses also welcomed the first patient to the institution that would be his home until he recovered or died. The unbalanced staff-to-patient ratio was temporary—all fifty beds in the new tuberculosis hospital were spoken for.[2]

Most of the first patients to populate the sanatorium were transfers from the City Hospital in Minneapolis. Once that migration was completed in April, others arrived from Thomas Hospital and University Hospital. Those institutions would continue to maintain isolation wards for tuberculous patients, but people with moderate or far-advanced tuberculosis would henceforth receive treatment in the sanatorium.[3]

Tuberculosis, commonly referred to as TB, is as old as civilization. In 460 B.C.E., Hippocrates identified "phthisis" as the most prevalent disease of his time.[4] A few doctors hypothesized as early as the eighteenth century that people could catch tuberculosis if they had significant contact with an infected person, but prevailing theories included hereditary predisposition and unconventional lifestyles. The deaths of famous writers, composers, and actors seemed to support a relationship between creativity and tuberculosis. Among those dying were Frederic Chopin, composer; Anton Chekov, playwright; Robert Louis Stevenson, writer; and members of the Brontë family. Poet Alexander Pope survived tuberculosis, but it caused him to be hunchbacked.

Tuberculosis is contagious, though, and spread primarily through the air via phlegm or sputum during a cough or sneeze. Its underlying cause remained unknown until improved magnification capabilities of the microscope enabled German physician Robert Koch to isolate and identify the rod-shaped bacillus, *Mycobacterium tuberculosis humanis*, in 1882.

The human body tries to protect itself from a tuberculosis infection by encapsulating the bacillus in a firm nodule called a tubercle so the germs cannot multiply elsewhere. If that process is completed, a person is considered to have arrested or latent tuberculosis and is not contagious. If immunity is compromised by overwork, poor nutrition, or other illnesses, bacteria can breech the capsule walls, and the disease is once again active.

A person who has tuberculosis is referred to as tuberculous, meaning that tubercles have formed as a result of the presence of the tubercle bacillus. Saying that a patient with tuberculosis is tubercular is not as accurate, because that word encompasses a variety of diseases that manifest nodes or tubers, including leprosy.[5]

If tuberculosis is in the lungs, the most frequent location, it is known as pulmonary tuberculosis. Because the lungs have no sensory nerve fibers to cause pain, the disease can be far advanced before diagnosis. Pulmonary TB was commonly called consumption for its tendency to slowly consume its victims, who would lose weight, become pale and waste away. Some forms acted more quickly and were described as "galloping consumption." The sufferers' pallor led to a popular description, "the white plague."

The disease can affect any part of the body, however, which complicates the process of diagnosis and treatment. Tuberculosis occurring outside the lungs is termed extra-pulmonary. It can be in the brain and any of the inner organs such as stomach and kidneys, as well as the spine, knee, hip, etc. About the only parts of the body that the tubercle bacillus can't infect are hair and nails.

Tuberculosis is not always fatal. Mortality records kept in the years before the advent of antibiotics and chemotherapy vary considerably in reliability, but they indicate that forty to fifty percent of people affected by tuberculosis would survive. Accuracy in record keeping was made difficult by the elapse of months or years between onset and death and by other complications, such as pneumonia.[6]

Tuberculosis receded into history as a major cause of death in the United States and other more developed countries by the mid-twentieth century, but it was never eradicated worldwide, as smallpox was. Because smallpox is a virus-caused infection, vaccination by inoculation was able to eradicate that disease.

Researchers sought a vaccination that could be as effective as that for smallpox. BCG (Bacillus of Calmette and Guerin, named after two researchers) was first introduced in France in 1913 as a tuberculosis vaccine for cattle. It never gained much use in the United States among veterinarians, primarily because health departments in this country encouraged tuberculin testing and herd control. Also, BCG's efficacy was unproven, with experiments producing wildly differing results. Its unreliability and side effects meant it was never widely used in the United States on people, either. BCG would be used occasionally as an immunizing agent for medical personnel or the children of parents with tuberculosis. It would make them a positive reactor to tuberculin, and theoretically at least, they would have greater protection against the bacilli.

Tuberculosis is a bacterial infection. Because the outer layer, or membrane, of the bacillus contains no blood vessels, it is difficult for medication to penetrate and destroy the bacteria. Streptomycin was developed in the 1940s and hailed as a wonder drug, but it produced severe side effects. Eventually, a combination of drugs was used to successfully attack the bacteria and provide a cure for tuberculosis.[7]

We don't know for certain if tuberculosis existed in Minnesota prior to white settlement. When traders and missionaries populated newly explored areas in the Americas and near the Pacific Ocean, quite often they found no evidence of tuberculosis or other contagious diseases. For the most part, Ojibwe and Dakota Native American tribes in Minnesota lacked domesticated herd animals, a source of many deadly microbes to which the explorers and missionaries had developed some resistance.[8] Writings by seventeenth-century Jesuits who explored the Great Lakes suggest there may have been a few cases of glandular and pulmonary tuberculosis among the natives, but they were so rare the priests assumed the disease had been imported by European settlers.[9]

Whether the post-contact prevalence of tuberculosis demonstrates a lack of immunity or is the result of reservation development is a continuing debate.[10] Anthropologist Paul Farmer believes the rise was "clearly linked to a rapid decline in their standard of living."[11] That change began after the Removal Act of 1830, when Indians started receiving government annuities and were more likely to exchange money with fur traders, instead of hunting for fur pelts.[12]

Unfortunately, the European immigrants erroneously perceived North America to be an area of immunity. Their reports about this disease-free Eden encouraged even more Europeans to follow them, thus spreading the tubercle bacillus widely among societies that lacked natural defenses. Reverend Samuel Pond, a missionary in Minnesota, wrote in 1834 that "except the diseases incident to infancy and childhood, the Dakota suffered more perhaps from scrofula and consumption than from any other diseases."[13] Although scrofula is a particular form of TB occurring in lymph nodes, the term was often used to describe all non-lung tuberculosis.

Minnesota created a battlefield for health in the mid-1800s through a series of promotional publications designed to lure travelers, invalids, and immigrants. The literature claimed that dysentery, malaria, typhoid fever, and cholera were practically unknown because of the state's location in the central part of the North American continent.[14] The influx of travelers increased, seduced by pamphlets and newspaper articles that emphasized Minnesota's outdoor assets and downplayed its temperamental weather.

J.W. McClung extolled the virtues of camping out on lakeshores and growing strong and robust in a "free, independent, and romantic style." His testimonials praised the "invigorating prairie breezes" and suggested that consumptive invalids should arrive in May and use the summer and fall months to prepare their system for the "rousing exhilaration of our zeros and forties below."[15]

One of the earliest eastern immigrants mentioned is Clara Tuttle, who taught in what might have been the first school in Minneapolis in 1851. She returned to her home back east the next summer and died of consumption.[16]

Dr. Brewer Mattocks noted that Minnesota had "a society superior to most of the new states, because many families of wealth and high social position are obliged to live in our state on account of ill health."[17] Several decades later, F. Scott Fitzgerald would agree, saying the second-generation Germans and Irish in St. Paul "became passionately 'swell' on its own account. But the pace was set by the tubercular Easterners."[18]

Hotels that catered to the needs of consumptive visitors prospered as the relatively affluent Easterners flocked here for improved health. Dr. Mattocks stated that Minnesota was "a state of hotels." St. Paul had three that were first-class: the Metropolitan, the Park Place Hotel, and the Merchants' Hotel. Minneapolis was credited as having one top-rate hotel, the Nicollet House. In addition, private boarding houses sprang up to accommodate the invalids at prices ranging from six to ten dollars a week per person.[19]

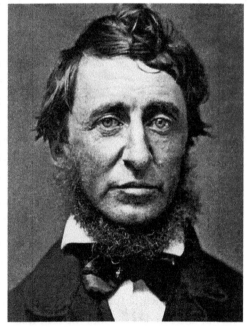

Henry David Thoreau, philosopher and poet, was told in 1861 that he should leave Concord, Massachusetts, and visit the West Indies or elsewhere to recover from what was referred to as bronchitis. Travel to other climates was regarded as healthy exercise and became a common prescription for people suffering from lung maladies. Thoreau decided against the West Indies, though, and sought instead the "air of Minnesota" in which to fight his consumption.[20]

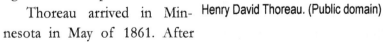

Henry David Thoreau. (Public domain)

Thoreau arrived in Minnesota in May of 1861. After spending several weeks in St. Paul, St. Anthony, and Minneapolis, he embarked on a steamboat excursion that traveled to Redwood and the Lower Sioux Agency in western Minnesota, where Native Americans who had arrived for a council with the governor's representatives were encouraged to dance for the travelers.[21] By August, Thoreau had returned to Concord, after a summer of seemingly constant traveling. In a letter to a friend he noted that his cough still continued, and he had been "sick so long that I have almost forgotten what it is to be well."[22] Thoreau died of tuberculosis on May 6, 1862.

The *Minnesota Guide* noted that a "very large proportion of the persons dying in the city [St. Paul] are strangers, who have come here sick and almost dying, to receive the benefits of our salubrious climate, but only to linger a few months and then cease the struggle. The city is constantly filled with them in all stages of disease."[23] Dr. William W. Mayo said, "Our state has become a large suburban hospital, receiving from every state of the Union invalids who are seeking relief from that fell destroyer, consumption . . ."[24] Mayo was himself a health seeker, fleeing from "the malarial hell of the Wabash Valley in Indiana."[25]

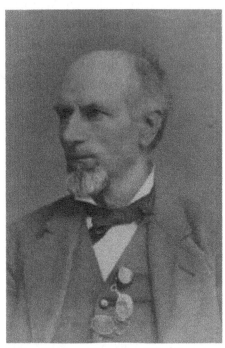

William W. Mayo. (Courtesy of the Olmsted Historical Society)

Eventually the southwestern states eclipsed Minnesota as a prime destination for consumptives, but tuberculosis had been invited, and it stayed. Its presence was helped by Scandinavian immigrants, who began arriving in large numbers. The 1850 census counted twelve Scandinavians in Minnesota; there were nearly 12,000 ten years later.[26] Unfortunately, a tuberculosis outbreak sweeping across Europe peaked in Norway and Sweden at about the time many of their citizens immigrated to Minnesota. Thus, the number of deaths attributed to tuberculosis continued to keep pace with population increases throughout the 1880s.[27]

The leaders of Minnesota's medical professions and public health boards were aware of the tuberculosis problem in the state. In 1870, the census in Minnesota counted a population of 439,706. That year, scrofulous diseases killed 553 people, with 445 of those identified as lung consumption. Only forty-eight of the 553 were born in Minnesota, so it was assumed that many of the other cases came to Minnesota already infected with the disease.[28] For the years 1887 through 1899, approximately 20,000 persons in Minnesota died of tuberculosis, averaging ten percent of all deaths over that period.[29]

Doctors in Minneapolis and St. Paul urged a sanitation campaign to act upon the discovery that tuberculosis was contagious. For them, "sanitation" referred to not only clean water and sewage, but the entire process of keeping places free from dirt, infection, and disease. That included the use of such measures as burning soiled handkerchiefs and bedding.

The sanitation drives sought to educate the populace about hygiene and the need to refrain from spitting on floors and sidewalks. The first ordinance in Minneapolis against "indiscriminate and careless spitting" was passed in 1897, but applied only to street cars. It was amended later that year to include public halls, buildings, and sidewalks. Another ordinance in 1904 expanded the prohibition to depots, markets, theatres, churches, or any place of public amusement. It also made spitting a misdemeanor and imposed a fine of five dollars. Active enforcement resulted in 239 arrests and fines that year.[30]

The medical community also discussed using quarantines to impress the populace with the idea that "tuberculosis is catching." Most doctors dismissed this approach. They believed that quarantines would not work because tuberculosis was not curable. Invalids might not seek care if a diagnosis of tuberculosis meant a sentence of isolation until death.[31]

Most people with tuberculosis were cared for at home by friends and family who shouldered the burden. The earliest tuberculosis organization in Minnesota, the Anti-Tuberculosis Association of Willmar, was formed in 1890 to assist with home care. One of the founders, Dr. Edward S. Frost, had recently moved to Minnesota from the East Coast. Willmar's volunteer group, supported by donations of food and money, constructed and distributed fresh-air hoods for windows. These allowed the patients to sit or lie by an open window in rainy weather or the winter without the rest of the household experiencing temperature extremes.[32]

County poor farms often took in tuberculous people, but the personal care was inconsistent and mostly inadequate. In many of those houses, little attempt was made to segregate them from other residents. Some isolation was provided in others. Robert Hall of Olmsted County reported in 1901 that when he first became a county commissioner, he arranged for an isolated room to house consumptives.[33]

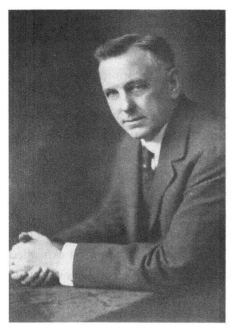

Henry Longstreet Taylor. (Courtesy of the Minnesota Historical Society)

A plan to care for tuberculosis patients at the Ramsey County Poor Farm in the 1890s backfired when Dr. Henry Longstreet Taylor provided tents to accommodate a few more invalids during the summer. The action was unpopular in the neighborhood when the tent colony spread to nearby fields. To prevent the tents from being pitched the next year, neighbors of the poor farm plowed the fields and planted potatoes.[34]

While the contagious nature of tuberculosis was beginning to be accepted, doctors had yet to agree on how to diagnose it. At the beginning of the twentieth century, many still relied on the presence or absence of specific symptoms such as fever, rapid pulse, blood spitting, excess sputum, and weight loss. Dr. John W. Bell claimed that auscultation (listening to breath sounds with a stethoscope) furnished the most important evidence. Very few doctors depended on a tuberculin test, which had been used in Europe since its discovery in 1890 by Dr. Koch. He initially thought an injection of heat-killed tubercle bacilli could cure tuberculosis. He was wrong, but the injection site manifested a reaction that was a relatively accurate indication of tuberculosis in a patient—either passive or active. The tuberculin test became generally known as the Mantoux after a French doctor refined the testing agent in 1907.[35]

There was no danger of contracting TB from the test, because the tuberculin contained only the protein of tubercle bacilli, which was injected into layers of skin, usually on a forearm. If the person had been previously infected, a swelling or allergic reaction appeared at the injection site. The diagnosis tool was important because by the time symptoms were obvious, tuberculosis was in an advanced state. The contagious person had most certainly infected someone else by the time they sought medical help and any chance of survival had been lessened.

The tuberculin test eventually gained favor among doctors for diagnosing tuberculosis. The number of new cases reported to the Minneapolis Health Department rose from less than 800 in 1910 to almost 1,200 in 1915. The rapid upswing was attributed to more accurate and earlier diagnoses rather than to increases in population or infections.

With the tuberculous population on the rise, physicians and families questioned where to house contagious patients. Early in the 1900s, some families erected tents and cabins in their backyards to provide isolation for an infected spouse or child. It must have been a special challenge for them to provide meals and to dispose of waste during a cold and snowy winter. Many hospitals were barely more than boarding houses. Few had the ability to isolate large numbers of people with such an infectious disease. Something had to be done, and the proposed solution was one that had gained popularity in Europe and the eastern United States: sanatoriums.

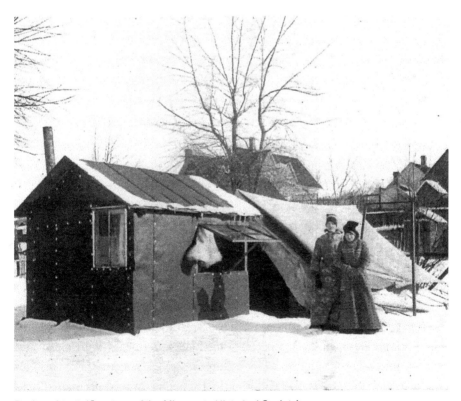

Backyard tent. (Courtesy of the Minnesota Historical Society)

2

Sanatoriums in Minnesota

HOSPITALS FOR PEOPLE WITH TUBERCULOSIS existed in Europe in the 1800s, but Dr. Hermann Brehmer is credited with popularizing the sanatorium concept. He believed that fresh air and a healthful climate were essential in the treatment of consumption, but that it was necessary to also include exercise and adequate nutrition. He established a tuberculosis sanitarium in Görbersdorf, Silesia, in 1854, and based it on his own successful health-seeking sojourn in the Himalayan Mountains.[1]

Thomas Mann used a similar sanatorium setting for his book *Magic Mountain*. His wife's illness and her stay at the Davos Sanatorium provided the backdrop for his commentary on society.[2]

Personal experience also prompted the establishment of what is generally recognized as the first tuberculosis institution in the United States. Its founder, Dr. Edward Livingston Trudeau, was well-acquainted with tuberculosis. As a young man in New York he cared for his older brother, James, who eventually died. Trudeau most likely contracted the disease himself from that ministry, much as the poet John Keats did in nursing his brother Tom. Trudeau sought a cure in Minnesota and spent the winter of 1873 in St. Paul. In keeping with medical theories of that era, he was allowed to walk and go duck hunting, even though experiencing a fever most of the time.[3]

Trudeau, feeling no improvement from his stay in Minnesota, returned to New York and traveled to the Adirondack Mountains. His hotel was without running water, but offered fresh and delicious meals, with clean and comfortable accommodations. His health improved, and the next summer he returned with his wife and children. In 1876, they moved permanently to the Adirondack village of Saranac Lake. In 1882, he learned about Brehmer's sanatorium and the work of Peter Dettweiler, who continued Brehmer's work but advocated rest instead of exercise. Trudeau embraced the concept of treating tuberculosis with fresh air, rest, and observation of the patient's daily life. By 1885, Trudeau welcomed the first two patients to his privately financed institution, known as the Adirondack Cottage Sanitarium.[4]

At that time, most institutions concerned with mental or physical health were known as sanitariums. By the turn of the century, the Canadian and American anti-tuberculosis associations wanted to distinguish between health resorts and the new type of hospital for tuberculosis. Instead of using the word sanitarium, which is derived from the Latin noun "sanitas," meaning "health," they emphasized the role of treatment in their institutions. In 1904, the associations formally approved using the word sanatorium, from the Latin verb root "sano," meaning "to heal."[5]

Most of the early sanatoriums, such as New York's Montefiore Home Country Sanatorium, were operated as privately funded non-profits. Others

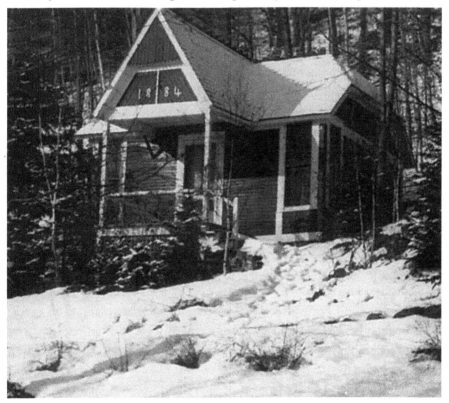

Little Red Cottage. (Public domain)

were affiliated with a religious organization, such as Gabriels Sanatorium in the state of New York. It was opened near Saranac Lake in 1895 by the Roman Catholic Sisters of Mercy and was named after Bishop Henry Gabriels.[6]

As the need grew for isolation of large numbers of infectious people, governmental entities debated the role of public funding and which of them should bear fiscal responsibility for building sanatoriums. Construction began on several state-supported sanatoriums. The first, Rutland State Sanatorium in Massachusetts, opened in 1898, with Dr. Walter Marcley as the first superintendent. By the early 1900s, several East Coast counties with large populations were building their own public sanatoriums and employing the Trudeau model of treatment in rural, wooded areas.

As part of a sanitation campaign in Minnesota, public health workers attempted to persuade the public that providing housing to those afflicted with tuberculosis was in their community's best interest. Bed rest, fresh air, and good food were really all they could offer patients in the early years, but it benefitted a community by isolating people to stop the spread of TB germs.

Dr. Henry Longstreet Taylor actively promoted the sanatorium concept as a solution to the increasing mortality rate due to tuberculosis. He had spent two years studying with Dr. Koch in Berlin and had practiced medicine at the Asheville Sanatorium in North Carolina before coming to Minnesota in 1893.[7] Taylor published "The Necessity of Special Institutions for the Consumptive Poor" in the *Northwestern Lancet* in that year, but his viewpoint was not widely supported by his fellow physicians at the time.[8]

In 1899, a report from the Minnesota Medical Association's Committee on Legislation noted Minnesota's efforts to create a national park and suggested that the northern part of the state would also offer an ideal setting for a sanatorium. The report mentioned successful sanatoriums in New York's Adirondack region and Georgia's pine forests as reasons to establish an institution near Cass or Leech lakes. Several men formed the Minnesota National Park and Forest Reserve Association, and they planned an excursion for members of Congress to the northern regions of Minnesota. The park project did not develop at that time, but the idea for a state sanatorium had been planted.[9]

A bill for the establishment of a state sanatorium was sponsored in the 1901 legislature. Midway during committee discussions, another bill was introduced that called for a commission to study the need and report to the next legislature. This second bill passed and was signed by Governor Samuel Van Sant. Dr. Taylor was appointed chair of the commission, which had the authority to select a site. The members visited many sanatoriums in the United States. They also scouted a number of potential locations in Minnesota, but noted that "many communities were stricken with acute phthisiophobia (fear of tuberculosis) upon the appearance of the commission in their midst."[10]

Commission members learned from their research that the ideal site would be close to a population center and railroads, but they understood that funding appropriations would be more likely if their choice was in northern Minnesota. Their final report listed their reasons for endorsing a state sanatorium to be built near Walker, by Leech Lake. Among the reasons was its location in the pine region near the Chippewa/Ojibwe reservation. It was in an area that had been logged and was being reseeded. The region was sparsely settled and, thus, lessened chances of contaminating an existing population. There was a good supply of pure water and an area large enough for a farm to support a dairy herd and vegetable gardens. The commission also claimed the location was not far north of the geographical center of the state. Unmentioned was the fact that it was 180 miles from the population centers of Minneapolis and St. Paul, a distance that in 1903 could prohibit many families and friends from visiting the patients.[11]

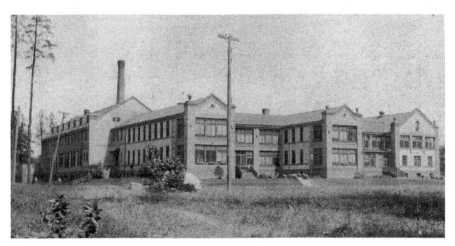

State sanatorium postcard. (Author's collection)

A bill from the 1903 legislature provided $25,000 to purchase 616 acres at ten dollars per acre near Walker. It was also enough to survey and grade the site, but not enough for construction. The 1905 legislature made a further appropriation of $50,000. Thus, with the delays caused by commission

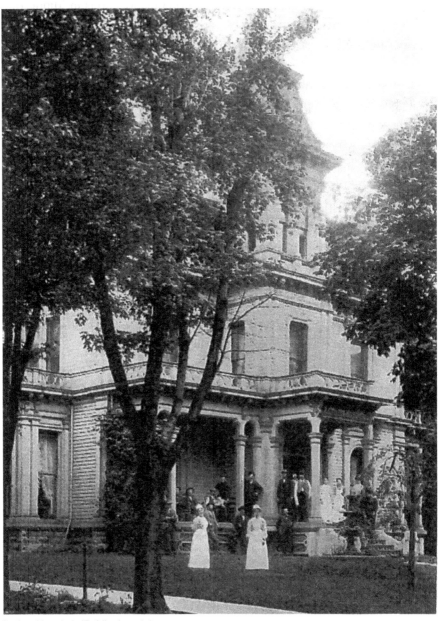

Luther Hospital. (Public domain)

reports and inadequate budgets, the Minnesota State Sanatorium for Consumptives did not open until December 27, 1907.

The sanatorium was placed under the management of Minnesota's Board of Control for State Institutions, which was responsible for prisons and mental hospitals. Dr. Marcley was appointed as superintendent. Shortly after its opening, the sanatorium was renamed "Ah-gwah-ching," an Ojibwe phrase meaning "out-of-doors." Ah-gwah-ching would eventually serve twenty-four counties in Minnesota that did not affiliate with a local sanatorium.[12]

While legislators were settling the issue of the state sanatorium, the spread of tuberculosis had continued. One person in particular, commission chair Taylor, chafed under the delays while the state pondered its response to the rising death toll. In 1902, he had worked with Dr. Eduard Boeckmann to establish a tuberculosis ward in Ancker Hospital in St. Paul. In 1903, he established a tuberculosis ward in Luther Hospital at John and Tenth streets. In 1905, he used his own money to open a private institution near Pine City, named Pokegama Sanatorium for its location on the lake of that name. In 1910, the doctor helped open Cuenca Sanatorium on Bass Lake and a summer camp for tuberculosis patients in White Bear Lake.[13]

Dr. Taylor wasn't the only one who had become impatient with the slow pace of the state's plan. George H. and Lenore Christian lost a son, Henry,

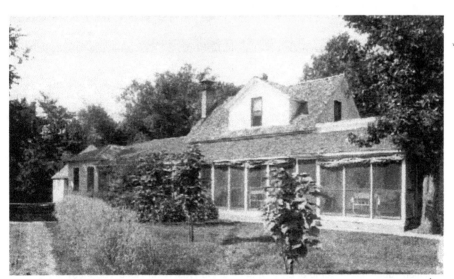

Pokegama Cottage. (Courtesy of the Minnestoa Historical Society)

to tuberculosis in 1905. Mr. Christian managed the Washburn flour mill in Minneapolis, and it was under his direction that the mill increased its production capacity. As a result, the Christians were among the wealthiest of Minnesotans. Henry had most likely contracted tuberculosis at Yale, where dormitories provided conditions that favored the spread of tuberculosis. Unlike many people of their social status who hid the presence of TB in their family, the Christians were motivated to combat the disease. They had the financial ability to support several initiatives through generous philanthropy.

In 1906, they opened the Christian Tuberculosis Camp on on Lake Street and Forty-sixth Avenue South, with twenty-two children registered. At this tent camp overlooking the Mississippi River upstream from St. Paul, some tuberculous adult patients lived year-round. During the summer, the children had their meals outdoors, rested on their cots or played, and received treatment for active tuberculosis. Mrs. Christian not only visited the camp daily, but she called upon the families of the children to offer needed assistance. The camp operated for two years.[14]

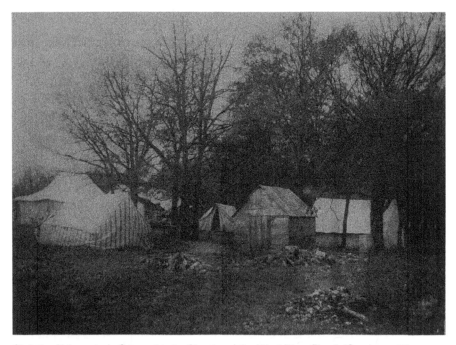

Christian Tuberculosis Camp at Lake Street and the West River Road. (Courtesy of the Minnesota Historical Society)

At the time, fourteen beds at City Hospital were the only provision for tuberculous patients in Minneapolis.[15] George Christian criticized the existing accommodations in the city, saying, "There are 2,000 cases of consumption in the city, and none of the hospitals except the City admits patients affected with tuberculosis, and at the City Hospital they are only accepted about two or three weeks before they die." In response, the couple personally financed the construction of a hospital at 2341 Sixth Street South.[16]

The facility opened as the Christian Memorial Hospital, but Mrs. Christian renamed it Thomas Hospital in memory of Bishop Thomas, former rector at St. Mark's Episcopal Church. Its operation was later turned over to the United Lutheran Church.[17] She is also given credit for convincing the city of Minneapolis that it needed additional TB beds, resulting in the construction of Hopewell Hospital in 1908, built on land donated by William Hood Dunwoody.[18] On opening day there were more applicants for admission than the capacity. Mrs. Christian also supported the local sales of Red Cross "holiday stickers" for one cent apiece. The stickers were affixed to mailed envelopes and gift packages and were popularly known as Christmas Seals.[19]

In 1909, more than 350 private and state tuberculosis sanatoriums were in operation in the United States. Only three were in Minnesota: Ah-gwah-ching, Pokegama, and Piney Ridge, which a doctor had established in small cabins on Big Whitefish Lake.[20] Because the distance to Ah-gwah-ching from the southern corners of the state was nearly 300 miles, county commissioners urged their legislative representatives to develop a plan for housing

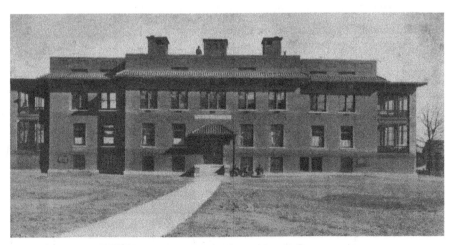

Thomas Hospital. (Courtesy of the Hennepin History Museum)

The building at the bottom center is the original sanatorium. (Courtesy of the University of Minnesota-Duluth Martin Library)

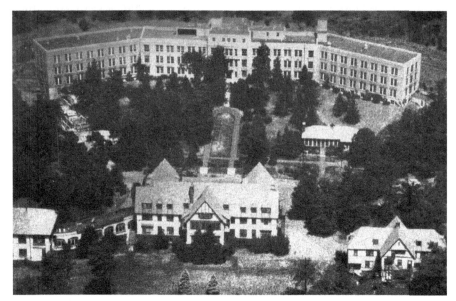

and treating people near their own homes. Although the 1909 legislature authorized counties to form districts, appoint boards, and build sanatoriums, it did not designate any state monies to be spent. Dr. Edward L. Tuohy guided the establishment of the first county sanatorium near Duluth in 1912. St. Louis County self-funded the construction of Nopeming, which is Ojibwe for "place of rest."

The 1913 legislature appropriated $500,000 to be used by counties as matching funds for construction. Counties responded quickly. By 1918, Minnesota had fourteen county sanatoriums, more per capita than any other state.

Sanatoriums in order of opening with member counties and original capacity

Name	County/ies served initially	Open	City	Capacity
Nopeming	St. Louis	1912	Nopeming	50
Otter Tail	Otter Tail	1913	Battle Lake	37
Ramsey	Ramsey	1914	St. Paul	110
Mineral Springs	Goodhue	1915	Cannon Falls	34
Glen Lake	Hennepin	1916	Oak Terrace	50
Sunnyrest	Norman, Polk	1916	Crookston	26

Name	County/ies served initially	Open	City	Capacity
Lake Julia	Beltrami, Hubbard, Itasca, Koochiching	1916	Puposky	25
Sand Beach	Becker, Clay	1916	Lake Park	26
Riverside	Chippewa, Lac qui Parle, Renville, Yellow Medicine	1917	Granite Falls	40
Buena Vista	Wabasha, Winona	1917	Wabasha	30
Southwestern	Cottonwood, Jackson, Lincoln, Lyon, Murray, Nobles, Pipestone, Rock	1917	Worthington	45
Oakland Park	Marshall, Pennington, Red Lake, Roseau	1918	Thief River Falls	25
Fair Oaks Lodge	Todd, Wadena	1918	Wadena	24
Deerwood	Aitkin, Crow Wing	1918	Deerwood	24

The Minnesota Sanatorium Advisory Commission assumed authority to establish the district sanatoriums, approve building plans, and set up rules and medical control. The state's Board of Health could approve only the water supply and sewage disposal plans because it had neglected to act on a state law of 1913, section 4640, giving it authority to establish broader regulations. County tuberculosis commissions were responsible for maintaining the institutions. A Minnesota State Board of Visitors charged with responsibility for examining the management and care of inmates in state institutions was assigned to study sanatoriums, too.

The overlapping and sometimes conflicting duties led to several disagreements. The Board of Health's director, Dr. Henry Bracken, expressed dissatisfaction with architectural plans approved by the Sanatorium Advisory Commission for several of the county institutions. Of the Wabasha sanatorium, he said that he was "letting the county sanatorium commission and the advisory commission have full credit for all of the mistakes, as we see them, on the plans for this county sanatorium." He also said that the plans for Lake Julia water supply were so bad that the board was not willing to approve them without a protest, but had no choice because construction was almost complete by the time they saw the plans.[21]

Regarding the design of several other sanatoriums, Bracken stated his belief that the additional expense of reinforced concrete floors and fire-proof construction put an unnecessary strain on county budgets. Glen Lake Sanatorium, in Hennepin County, was built to those specifications anyway. It was to become not only the largest sanatorium in Minnesota, but one of the most prominent in the United States.

3

The First Year

A T THE TIME OF GLEN LAKE SANATORIUM'S construction, members of
the Hennepin County commission were Dr. John W. Bell, Joseph R.
Kingman, and Edward C. Gale.[1] The formal opening had been planned for
late in January 1916, but the commissioners advocated the early opening on
the sixth. They thought patients would be better off in a partially completed building than in their homes where they had "become a menace to the
health of others."[2] They were right to worry. The number of people dying
from tuberculosis kept pace with the population growth in Minneapolis and
increased from 273 in 1910 to 416 in 1915.[3]

Dr. Bell, a member of the original medical faculty at the University
of Minnesota and deeply involved in tuberculosis studies, was nevertheless a curious choice for commission membership. In 1890, Bell countered
Koch's finding of the bacillus with a theory of predisposition or heredity
rather than contagiousness. In 1909, he advocated keeping consumptives in
their own homes and relying on family physicians. Because of his teaching
background and his service as president of the State Medical Association in
1905, he influenced others. In his book *Invited and Conquered*, Dr. J.A. Myers
goes so far as to say that there is "little doubt that his [Bell's] statements
checked progress toward the development of institutions for the tuberculous."[4]

Mr. Kingman was a prominent Minneapolis attorney employed at the
Woods and Hahn law firm. By the time he retired in 1950, it was known as
the Kingman Firm. Mr. Gale was an attorney in the law firm of Snyder &
Gale. His wife, Sadie Belle, was the daughter of John S. Pillsbury, founder of
a grain processing company.

Because Minnesota was late in entering the sanatorium phase of tuberculosis treatment, several guides already existed to assist the commission members in planning. The National Association for the Study and Prevention of Tuberculosis had compiled a popular book titled *Tuberculosis Hospital and Sanatorium Construction*, which was into its third edition by 1914.[5] Its author, Dr. Thomas Spees Carrington, also wrote *Fresh Air and How to Use It*. His book about sanatoriums included the cost of construction, noting, "the problem of tuberculosis from the institutional point of view is to care for the largest possible number of patients at the lowest possible cost compatible with efficient result."

Nationally, patient demographics had slowly changed from wealthy Eastern cure seekers to low- and middle-class laborers. Tuberculosis became linked more often to poverty and sweatshops than to creativity and artistry. Many people lost their means of support due to their illness and lived in boarding houses or cold-water flats. They would depend on the county or state to pay for a portion of their care. Carrington said that a building constructed in a comparatively inexpensive manner with simplicity and economy would return patients to their homes "without making them unduly discontented with the environment and life to which they belong."[6] A sanatorium was not yet seen as having a role in any type of economic or social rehabilitation, but only as a last-chance place to conquer TB.

In the absence of strong commitment laws, Minnesota's new sanatoriums needed to be comfortable and attractive enough to entice patients to remain. The Glen Lake Sanatorium's location followed recommendations for placement on the southern exposure of a hill in an area of natural beauty to help "amuse patients and keep them contented."[7] The sanatorium commission members selected a site in the western end of the county in Minnetonka Township, about twelve miles from Minneapolis. The area, known as Little Switzerland, provided an expansive view of hills, marshes, and woods. It had been considered as the setting for a sanatorium as early as 1907, along with locations near the city of Savage and Christmas Lake near Chanhassen, when W.H. Dunwoody offered to buy land for that purpose.[8]

The mailing address for the new sanatorium was Hopkins, but the nearest population center was Glen Lake, a named neighborhood in the township. It had streetcar service, but the three-quarter-mile walk to the sanatorium from the station at Eden Prairie Road and Excelsior Boulevard was an inconvenience for employees and visitors until a wagon and a white horse were purchased to transport people to and from the streetcar. The driver, named Andrew, converted the wagon wheels to sleigh runners in the winter.[9] Ambulance service for patients was initially provided by the City Hospital of Minneapolis.[10]

The sanatorium took its name from the settlement and a nearby lake, which were named after the first registered owners, Robert Glen and his wife, Mary, who purchased land in 1857. The undeveloped property passed through several owners, including John Chastek, before being bought by the county. One of the land speculators named on the deed in 1863 was Susan Damon Gale, wife of Samuel C. Gale and mother of commission member Edward.[11] The sanatorium was also situated on land served by the spur of a railroad line, important for the delivery of coal to run the power plant that produced steam heat and electricity. The sanatorium's first buildings followed a simple design recommended by Carrington's guide. The commissioners forwent the wood-frame buildings with open porches, known as King Lean-tos, that were popular in states with more temperate climates. The first Hopewell Hospital had been built in that style, but it became evident that the extremes of Minnesota's weather demanded a substantial, permanent building.

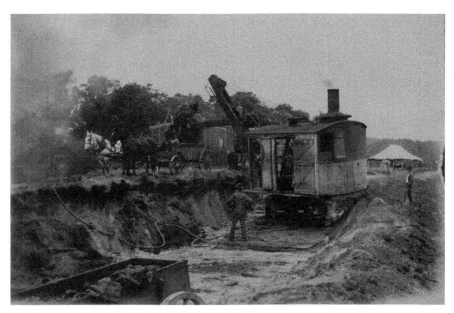

Construction. (Courtesy of the Minnesota Historical Society)

The architectural plans called for a pleasing symmetry of four rectangular structures built into the south slope of the hill, protecting the sanatorium from the north winds. Three buildings were to be placed in a slight arc in front of the fourth, the power plant, to hide it from full view. Construction started in 1914, with horses providing much of the power for grading and hauling. A coal-fired steam shovel carved into the hillside and excavated for the foundations.

The state of Minnesota and Hennepin County each contributed half the $100,000 cost of building the sanatorium, but that wasn't enough to complete the full plan. As a result, on opening day in 1916, the sanatorium consisted of an unbalanced arrangement of only three stucco craftsman-style buildings. The east, south, and west walls of the patients' building featured many windows reaching from floor to ceiling to allow ventilation. Screened areas on the south side had space for patients to sit in canvas cure chairs. One large tent provided additional fresh-air space.[12]

The two-story buildings were referred to as cottages, patterned after Trudeau's one- or two-bedroom accommodations at Saranac Lake. In contrast, Glen Lake's East Cottage contained forty beds in large rooms called wards. Women were on the first floor, men on the second. The *Tuberculosis Hospital and Sanatorium Construction* publication noted that most sanatoriums

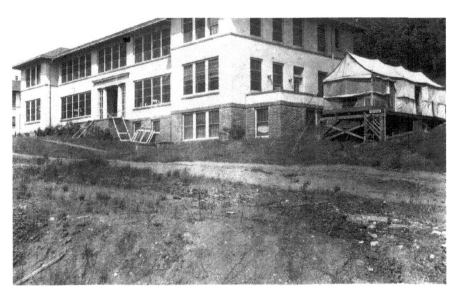

East Cottage with tent. (Courtesy of the Hopkins Historical Society)

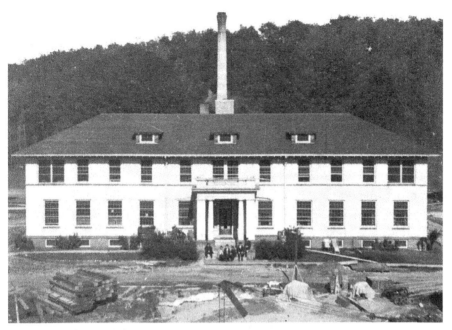

Administration cottage. (Courtesy of the Hopkins Historical Society)

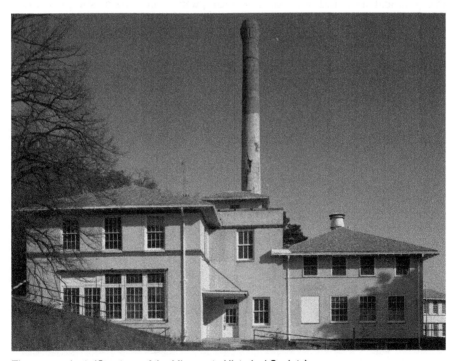

The power plant. (Courtesy of the Minnesota Historical Society)

segregated male and female and white and "colored" patients by floors, wards, or separate buildings.[13] Patients were not separated by race at Glen Lake, partly because the population served was predominantly white. The first black person, Leon Nichols, was not admitted until November.[14]

The accommodations for each patient consisted of an iron bed and a plain enameled metal bedstand. The sparse furnishings were indeed a function of the aforementioned "simplicity and economy." They were also easy to disinfect, a necessity when housing people with a contagious disease.

The middle or Administration Cottage housed the offices and reception room, the doctors' laboratory, an operating room, the drugstore, living quarters for the medical director and nurses, the main kitchen and bakery, and storerooms. It also could accommodate ten of the sanatorium's capacity of fifty patients. Most of the food was cooked in the administration kitchen and delivered to the East Cottage in custom-made carriers. Special-diet kitchens were located on each floor of the cottage.

The power plant building, tucked into the hill, generated electrical power and steam heat for the complex. It also contained living quarters for non-medical staff and housed the laundry, which had one washer, two ironing boards, and a flatwork ironer.

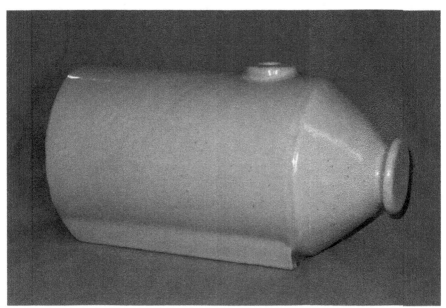

The pig warmer. (Author's collection)

26

When the sanatorium opened, Gertrude Moore was both the head nurse and the head of housekeeping. The staffing organization soon changed, and the nursing and housekeeping departments were separated.[15] Lucille Townsend came to Glen Lake as the director of household on September 1. The first food order she placed was with a local farmer for eight pounds of butter, three pecks of potatoes, and one peck of carrots.[16]

Glen Lake provided the basics of rest, fresh air, and good food. It's unlikely that the sanatorium's first patients completely understood what was in store for them concerning the part about rest. From the time Glen Lake opened in 1916 until the widespread use of chemotherapy in the 1950s, the average length of a stay was rarely less than two years.[17] Patients spent months in bed in an open ward. Television didn't exist. Personal radios and phonographs were too expensive for most patients to own. The shared bathroom was down a hall, and patients weren't allowed to use it until the doctor gave permission. Climate control consisted of the windows, which were open year-round so patients could have daily exposure to fresh air. Winter nights often demanded hibernation under several woolen blankets. Summer air conditioning was a fan.

A March 12, 1916, article in the *Minneapolis Morning Tribune* reported that several Glen Lake patients were spending time on the porch.

> It was a cold day and there was a sharp wind, but the men and women patients, in their separate wards, had their beds wheeled out to the porch and, securely blanketed, lay there drinking in the pure air that came through the wide-open windows. A few held papers in their mittened hands, but the majority chatted with their neighbors or lay with closed eyes, resting.

The article noted there were more men admitted than women. When the reporter asked who was the oldest patient, a nurse said she didn't know, but a "gray-haired old lady popped her head up from her pillow. 'Guess I am,' she remarked, evidently eager for the honor. 'I'm fifty-seven.' 'I guess you're right, Mother Kelly,' smiled the nurse. 'And our youngest patient is Dolly, aged sixteen.'"[18]

In addition to the woolen blankets, the patients had "pigs" to keep them warm. The stoneware pottery jugs were filled with hot water and tucked under

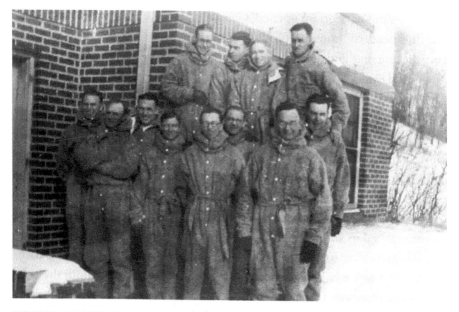

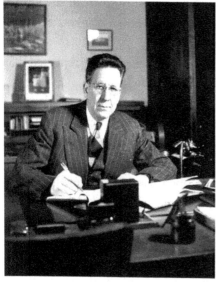

Sleeping suits. (Courtesy of the Lokke Collection)

Dr. Mariette (at left). (Courtesy of Hennepin History Museum)

blankets near the feet. The containers were called pigs because from the side looked like they had a snout. Some hardy residents of the East Cottage wore custom-sewn sleeping suits that covered them from head to toe so they could sleep on the porch all winter.[19]

Patients also employed a sleep-preparation technique described by Oletta Desmond:

When we went to bed, we really dressed. Usually we wore underwear, nightgowns, sweaters, caps, bathrobes, and very often, stockings and mittens. It was not unusual for a patient to have from twenty to twenty-five blankets on his bed. We made our beds Klondike style, which means putting one blanket crosswise in order to keep the others from pulling loose; and, of course, with this arrangement we had to slide into them from the top.[20]

Dr. Frank Jennings, who came to Glen Lake in 1917, said, "Sleeping out of doors at thirty degrees below zero was certainly no fun for the patients or for the doctor who not only had to enforce it but had to set an example by sleeping out himself." When not sleeping near the patients, doctors Jennings and Mariette had warmer rooms over the bakery.[21]

Accommodations at publicly funded Glen Lake differed from those at Pokegama Sanatorium, Dr. Taylor's private institution near Pine City. An advertisement for Pokegama in a 1915 Minneapolis directory touts the availability of electric blankets that "make outdoor sleeping in Minnesota comfortable."[22]

Sanatoriums also differed in how they handled the issues of contagion. At Glen Lake, the doctors wanted certain habits to become second nature to the patients, so they were expected to cover their noses and mouths when talking or sneezing. The philosophy at Glen Lake was that patients, when discharged, were responsible for themselves and also for safeguarding the health of others. They needed to learn good habits. Research in 1898 had shown that hands carried the greatest contamination, so handkerchiefs were replaced by folded gauze and paper napkins, which were burned. Disposable tissue wouldn't become available until introduced by the Kimberly-Clark Company in 1924, and it would be in the mid-1930s before patients had access to a paper tissue that was soft and came in a dispenser. Glen Lake patients were also provided with waxed paper sputum cups for expectoration.[23]

The doctors and nurses were gowned but not always masked. They washed hands and took precautions. At Ah-gwah-ching State Sanatorium, in contrast, even floor maids and people in dietary departments were required to wear masks.[24]

Although the patients were afflicted with a contagious disease, not all of them were incapacitated. For those who were mentally alert, merely resting and keeping warm were not sufficient activities to pass the time. Dr. Mariette appealed to the *Minneapolis Morning Tribune* readers for contributions of books and magazines. He mentioned that a Victrola or a piano would "help to while away many of the hours that often hang heavily."[25] His request drew a quick response. Twelve days later, the newspaper reported,

Glen Lake Sanatorium seemed like "home, sweet home" to the patients who are confined there. Music and reading matter to satisfy the most insatiable appetite for melody and literature were to be had for the asking. It was all the result of the arrival of a talking machine with about sixty-five records.

Mr. J.R. Byers, a cashier at the Minnesota Loan and Trust Company, had created a fund and named it "The Glen Lake Sanatorium Talking Machine Fund, Unlimited." He gathered donations from more than 100 individuals. A dry goods company provided the talking machine at a low cost, and several people contributed records. The Park Avenue Transfer Company delivered those, as well as several magazines and books.[26] The gifts marked the beginning of a long history of community involvement with the sanatorium.

Several human interest stories about the sanatorium appeared in the Minneapolis papers. One article introduced *Tribune* readers to Mr. William Pugsley, a silhouette artist. During his period of inactivity at Glen Lake in 1916, he cut animals, landscapes, and people out of black paper, which he would paste on a white background for the amusement for his children, described as "chubby, blue-eyed four-year-old Lawrence, and solemn-faced, brown-eyed seven-year-old Charlie, as they clambered about on his porch bed." Because he wasn't considered an active or contagious case, his children could visit him. Both Mr. and Mrs. Pugsley served as examples to the public that patients could be healed with only rest, fresh air, and good food. They contracted TB in their thirties, recovered their health, and lived into their sixties.[27]

The Pugsleys were among the fortunate. Most of the thirty-seven patients admitted in January came with diagnoses of "far advanced." Eleven would eventually die at the sanatorium. Two died that month, including first patient Andrew Gibson on the nineteenth. Ten people left against the advice of their physician, for reasons unrecorded but probably related to the stringent routine, boredom, or distance from their families. Toby Kleinbaum was one who left; she had a husband and two young children at home. She survived tuberculosis and had three more children. Aurelia Devereaux was also one of those who left, but she returned in July and stayed a year before being discharged. She lived another twenty-two years.[28] A search of death certificates for others who left revealed that many of them died within two years of leaving Glen Lake.

As patients left and empty beds became available, they were filled. The new sanatorium was already too small to meet the need. The Hennepin County Sanatorium Commission pushed for the construction of that other fifty-bed cottage to be located on the west side of the Administration Cottage. It had been included in the original layout and would balance the institution's appearance and increase the capacity to one hundred beds. The commission members requested a funding levy of $30,000 from the county commissioners in August 1916.

An impassioned opinion piece in the *Minneapolis Morning Tribune* called for the city's best thought and best effort in the "fight against the white terror." The war raging in Europe, which the United States had yet to join, likely influenced the paper's eloquent plea for additional beds.[29]

> Some of the trenches and battlements have been taken. The end is not in sight but there is progress. Here and there the host of the destroyer has been thrust back. If we put on the right kind of armor, equip ourselves with the proper weapons and keep strong in the faith of final victory we shall win some day. . . . It is a war of economics, of conservation, of humanity. From every viewpoint it is a war that calls for loyal, earnest soldiers under able generals.[30]

Dr. Collins, who was also the superintendent of the Minneapolis City Hospital, resigned as administrator at Glen Lake in August. Dr. Marcley had already returned to his previous affiliation with Hopewell Hospital. In September, Dr. Mariette accepted the appointment as superintendent and medical director at Glen Lake Sanatorium.

Ernest Sidney Mariette was relatively young to be given the responsibility, having received his Doctor of Medicine degree just three years earlier. He was a native Minnesotan, born in Good Thunder in 1888 to Sidney Brewer Mariette and his wife, Grace L. Garvin. They lived for a short time in the Blue Earth area and in South Dakota, where another son, Percy, was born. The family moved to a house at 2817 Fremont in Minneapolis, where Sidney Mariette worked for Van Dusen-Harrington, a grain processing and distribution business. Sidney passed away in 1906 from a pancreatic hemorrhage at the age of forty-one. The sons attended school in the Minneapolis Central District and completed their education at the Pillsbury Academy, a private school in Owatonna. They attended the University of Minnesota, and Ernest received his medical degree in 1913.[31]

Dr. Mariette served his residency at Nopeming Sanatorium and completed an internship at the University of Minnesota's hospital before coming to Glen Lake for its opening day. A colleague described him as a "solid man with a somewhat leonine head, who yet moves about rapidly. An energetic, decisive man, a man of action. One word description: vigorous."[32]

The facility that he assumed responsibility for, although recently built, was already outmoded and inadequate for the needs of tuberculosis patients. As its new supervisor, he began implementing his vision of an institution that addressed a broad spectrum of patients' needs, both clinical and non-clinical. In the phraseology of a later time, his approach would be called holistic. Glen Lake Sanatorium had found its "able general" in the person of its young administrator.

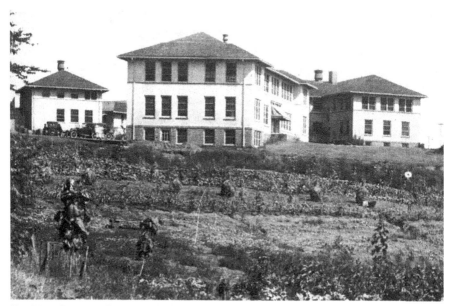

The West Cottage. (Courtesy of the Hopkins Historical Society)

4

More Space Needed

THE FUNDING REQUEST SUBMITTED by the sanatorium commissioners was reconsidered, and the Hennepin County commissioners provided $25,000 from tax revenues. In 1917, the West Cottage finally opened, with fifty more patients to feed and care for. The kitchen added an electric mixer. Food and dishes continued to be sent to the cottages in express carts and wooden boxes, and the laundry added two rollers to the flatwork ironer.[1]

With the addition of the West Cottage, the patient population at the sanatorium numbered 100. The charge for care was set by the state. Treatment cost seven dollars per week for residents who could pay and was offered free to indigent residents of the county, with five dollars of state aid paid to the sanatorium. Residents of other counties paid ten dollars per week. Because preference was given to Hennepin County residents, for whom there was always a waiting list, only non-residents with exceptional needs were accepted at Glen Lake. Patients who didn't wish to be in a public sanatorium and could afford to pay for greater privacy had the option of receiving care at Pokegama Sanatorium near Pine City. Weekly rates there ranged from twenty-two dollars and fifty cents for a bed in a ward to thirty-five dollars for a single occupancy cottage.[2]

Physicians and nurses at Glen Lake, in addition to providing medical care, also assisted patients with personal problems and attempted to alleviate their boredom. There was little precedent for understanding how patients coped with the prospect of living in a hospital bed for an extended amount of time. It was especially challenging for tuberculous patients, who didn't always feel seriously ill or in pain. With doctors unable and unwilling to set

deadlines for healing and discharge, sanatorium patients were voluntarily incarcerated without a defined sentence.

Managing this uncertainty and filling the long blocks of inactivity required more intervention than the doctors and nurses could perform.

Louis Grenier, a patient, came up with a solution to one problem. In
1917, retail stores in Hopkins and Minneapolis did not make deliveries to a
sanatorium located so far from them. With help from friends, Grenier began
operating a store out of suitcases, from which he sold magazines, pencils,
paper, and other items to fellow patients. Grenier spent many years at the
sanatorium. He was released in 1925 to continue his cure at home, but returned for a short time in 1930.[3]

The magazines, phonograph, and writing supplies helped to pass the
time, but more was needed. The Anti-Tuberculosis Committee within the
Associated Charities of Minneapolis took an interest in patient welfare and
agreed to pay the salary and expenses of a social worker until the sanatorium
could assume the additional expense. The committee described this as an
experiment, even though the first professional social worker had been hired
at Massachusetts General Hospital in 1905. The practice had already spread
to many other hospitals. Dorothy Walton came to Glen Lake as Minnesota's
first sanatorium social worker in February 1918.[4]

Also in 1918, instructors at the University of Minnesota's School of
Nursing began sending student nurses to Glen Lake to gain experience with
tuberculosis. The new faces were most likely a welcome diversion for the
socially isolated patients.

The conflict in Europe started to affect the sanatorium's operation. On
February 3, 1917, the United States broke diplomatic ties with Germany. On
April 6, it declared war. After the Selective Service Act was passed, thousands
of Minnesota recruits were processed through Fort Snelling, creating labor
shortages. Glen Lake operated as simply as possible and used cost-saving
measures. Planks on sawhorses were used for cafeteria tables, and trays were
borrowed from the YWCA.[5] Miss Walton resigned as social worker in 1919
in order to go to France and work among refugees from the Great War. She
was succeeded by Lanore Ward, who assumed the duties of a position still
described as an experiment. Her task was largely that of "infusing a cheery
community spirit into what would otherwise be a somewhat monotonous
round of treatments, rest, and exercise."[6]

One of Ward's efforts brought the outside world to the patients via moving pictures. The first show was a mixture of education and frivolity provided by Oscar Alm of the Anti-Tuberculosis Committee. A movie titled *Oral Health* and another about open-air schools in Chicago were followed by several short comedies, including *Missing Husbands* and *The Royal Nymphs*. Bed patients were wheeled from their wards into the large sitting rooms of each cottage to see the silent films.[7]

In 1919, Dr. Bell resigned from the Hennepin County Sanatorium Commission. He was replaced by Dr. Solon Marx White, whose involvement in combating tuberculosis included membership on the first medical committee that worked with the Christian family. He joined the University of Minnesota faculty in 1898 and was chairing its department of medicine at the time he became a member of the commission.[8]

The Great War played a role in the increased demand for tuberculosis care. Even though approximately 50,000 tuberculous men were rejected for service in the United States at the time of induction, thousands of soldiers were infected with TB during the war.[9] Dr. C.E. Banks, chief medical adviser of the Bureau of War Risk Insurance in Washington, D.C., informed the Minnesota State Board of Health that about 200 soldiers and sailors from the state had been discharged from service because of tuberculosis. Dr. Banks requested that the Board of Health cooperate in solving the problem of securing sanatorium treatment for those cases wherever home treatment was not advisable or was unsatisfactory.[10]

The first two of the expected Great War veterans arrived at Glen Lake in March 1919. Dr. Mariette was notified of their impending arrival by telegram from the bureau, which was paying the expense of treatment. This situation strengthened the argument for expansion of sanatoriums throughout Minnesota. Some believed that Glen Lake, even when enlarged to include additional beds, would not be sufficient to serve both civilian and soldier needs.[11] By 1922, more than 36,600 living veterans in the United States applied for service-connected tuberculosis compensation.[12] The Veterans' Administration Hospital in Minneapolis would not be built until 1927. Between 1919 and 1927, the Thomas Hospital was used by the U.S. government as a Veterans' Bureau Hospital.[13]

Concern for the patients' health and well-being extended beyond the life-threatening tuberculosis. Many arrived with additional medical issues, including heart disease, hyperthyroidism, gastrointestinal disturbances, and syphilis. The dental services required by Glen Lake's increasing number of patients led to the hiring of an in-house, full-time dentist in 1920. Dr. James C. Bryant graduated from the School of Dentistry of the University of Minnesota that year and almost immediately was employed at the sanatorium.[14]

Social worker Ward was also the director of occupational therapy. The craft work of patients at both Glen Lake and Hopewell Hospital was exhibited in April 1920 on the fourth floor of Donaldson's department store in Minneapolis. About 400 items were displayed, with the intent of demonstrating how handicrafts could help relieve the monotony of sanatorium life and consequently hasten recovery. Patronesses of the exhibit included Carolyn (Mrs. George C.) Christian, Mabel (Mrs. Joseph) Kingman, and Helen (Mrs. Sumner Jr.) McKnight.[15]

Another exhibit in December offered items for sale and was held at the Women's Club at 1726 Harmon Place in Minneapolis. Funds from the sale of such handmade articles as scarves, lamp shades, necklaces, and toys were shared by the individual patient and the sanatorium, to make the arts-and-crafts projects self-supporting. Although the contagiousness of tuberculosis was by now commonly known, there appears to have been no fear of transmission via these items sold.

In December 1920, Ward initiated a patients' newsletter known as *The Arrow*. This publication delivered news, gossip, and medical information.[16] Only five copies were produced, and one was given to each ward to share. Each front cover featured an original photo.[17]

The May 1921 issue (number six) listed the behaviors expected from people on the cure:

We are here to restore our health if possible.
To learn how to live regularly.
To learn how to protect ourselves and others around us.
To learn how to take care of ourselves.
To obey and ask no questions.
To take the cure faithfully; it is for our own good.
To respect the Doctors and Nurses as they do respect us.[18]

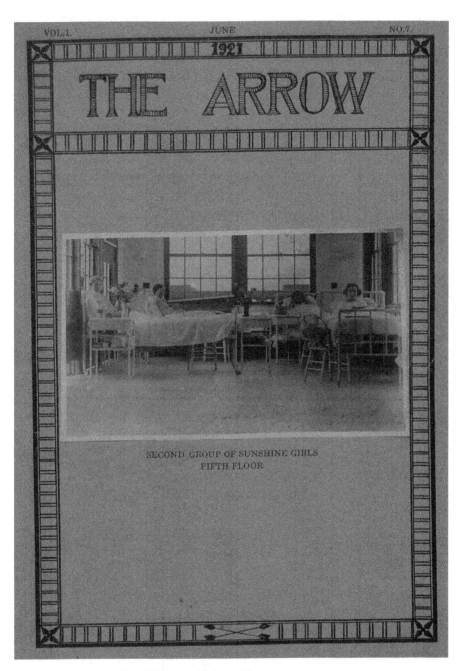

The Arrow. (Courtesy of the Minnesota Historical Society)

The "Current News" section reported that Dr. Mariette was attending a meeting of the National Tuberculosis Association and from there would be attending a six-week post-graduate course at the Trudeau School for Tuberculosis at Saranac Lake, New York. The school was founded by Dr. Edward Baldwin in 1916, in order to instruct physicians worldwide in the latest methods for treating tuberculosis.[19] The seventh issue of *The Arrow*, dated June 1921, was the last.

The Christmas holidays provided another opportunity for the social worker to produce that cheery community spirit she was charged with creating. In many hospitals and sanatoriums, it was customary to decorate and provide special treats and favors with a Christmas dinner. Ward worked with the Hennepin County Tuberculosis Association to augment that with a small Christmas tree for the bedside of each patient at Glen Lake, in addition to a large tree in the administration building. A concert program was presented on Christmas Eve, and the Good Fellowship class of Calvary Baptist church came on Christmas Day night to entertain.[20]

The staff at Glen Lake incorporated into the treatment plan whatever methods or tools might increase a patient's chances for a cure, but the capacity of the sanatorium was never enough to serve the need. All 100 beds were always full, and the waiting list never shortened. To meet the needs of the many people who remained on waiting lists, a request had been placed before the legislature in 1917 to add twenty-five beds at Hopewell Hospital and to construct an entire building at Glen Lake Sanatorium.

Dr. Pearl Hall, who wrote a health column for a daily newspaper, justified the $300,000 cost to house an additional 225 to 250 patients by pointing out that the only way to gain control over the disease was to isolate the advanced infectious cases. He saw the proper care of people with tuberculosis as an economic problem as well as one of health. "Poverty and tuberculosis go hand in hand," he said. "The community owes it to these unfortunate members of society to care for them properly."[21] The funding request was also endorsed by Dr. H.M. Guilford, head of the Minneapolis Department of Health, and Robley D. Cramer, editor of the *Minneapolis Labor Review*.[22]

Kathryne Radebaugh, education secretary of the Hennepin County Tuberculosis Association, commented on the continuing lack of room in TB facilities:

There is a family, including the parents and two children, all of them affected by tuberculosis. What we should like to do is to have them together at Glen Lake, but the room is not to be had. They cannot speak English to any extent—and it would be best to have them together as it would be possible for greater improvement to be realized in their condition.

Radebaugh said patients regarded Hopewell Hospital with a "rather chill feeling" and saw it not as a place to go for cure but rather as a place to die.[23]

Approval for enlargement of the sanatorium came in December 1918, and the new infirmary building formally opened on April 22, 1921. It was smaller than requested, increasing capacity by only 144 patients at a cost of $250,000. The contract was awarded to S.M. Klarquist & Son, with Sund & Dunham as the architects.[24]

Officials in attendance at the opening were entertained with a cartoon and moving pictures. The silent films featured the sanatorium and its method of cure and showed Governor Jacob Preus signing the sanatorium bond issue bill.[25]

The infirmary building was an impressive addition to the sanatorium campus. It was the first sanatorium in the U.S. to be taller than three stories, and four of its six floors were dedicated to patient care.[26] Its construction of reinforced concrete and brick made it fire-resistant.[27] About fifty beds remained in one of the cottages, which had been repurposed to house patients

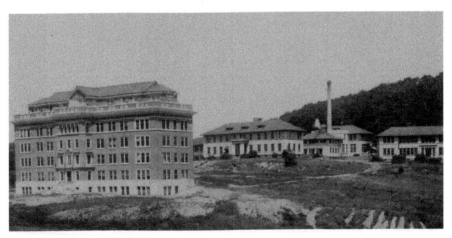

Infirmary construction. (Courtesy of the Minnesota Historical Society)

preparing for discharge. The other cottage was remodeled to provide living space for additional staff.

The infirmary's placement took advantage of the hill's south-facing slope and resulted in the top stories being level with the cottages farther up the hill. Two foundational levels—exposed to view only on the south side—housed medical and therapeutic services. The deck house and balcony configuration that crowned the building made it resemble an ark, while the roof of clay barrel tiles suggested a Spanish Mission lineage.

The building was built mostly for functionality, not style. The interior featured durable surfaces that could withstand frequent cleaning and disinfecting. Marble window sills were impervious to rain. Marble baseboards and terrazzo flooring tolerated mops and a dust-reducing compound consisting of paraffin oil and fine sawdust. Marble stall dividers complemented tiled walls in the bathrooms. Doorways were wide enough to allow patients to be moved while lying in beds and litters. In some rooms, the bottom sashes of triple-hung windows were flush with the floor. With the entire window raised, the patients could be wheeled onto the open porches in their own beds.[28]

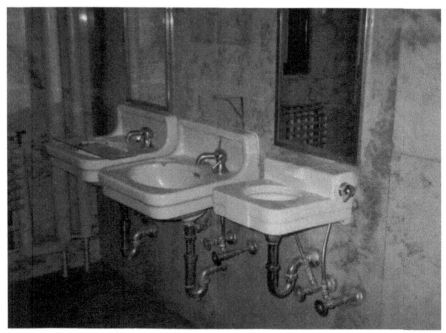

: Infirmary bathroom with special spit sink at right. (Courtesy of the Barker Collection)

The new hospital-type infirmary building meant more than just a doubling of available beds. Dr. Mariette strongly advocated for the continuing education of medical professionals. Dr. Marx, a member of the sanatorium commission and the University of Minnesota faculty, agreed and inaugurated an affiliation with the university's medical school. Future doctors were required to reside at the sanatorium for internships that included diagnostic, therapeutic and postmortem work. The university's nursing students served a six-week rotation in order to receive their diploma.[29] Other nursing schools and hospitals began requiring TB internships, and Glen Lake soon had students from Deaconess and Hillcrest in Minneapolis, from St. Olaf in Northfield, and even students from Miles City, Montana; Aberdeen, South Dakota; and schools in Canada.[30]

In 1921, for the first time, tuberculosis was no longer the leading cause of death in the United States. Heart disease had surpassed it, but that knowledge likely had little effect on the daily activities at Glen Lake Sanatorium. The busy sanatorium accommodated about three hundred people each day, thanks to the doubled patient population and increased staffing.

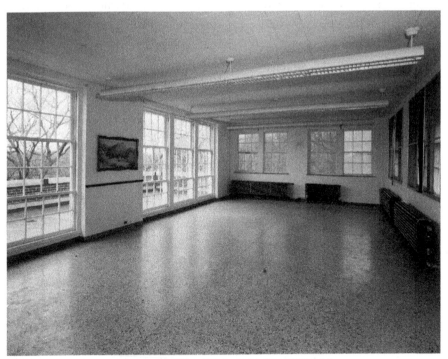

Infirmary windows. (Library of Congress, HABS MINN, 27 MINKA, 1J)

5

The Healing Sun

THE DESIGN OF THE NEW INFIRMARY BUILDING subtracted one element of the standard trinity of care—fresh air—and added a new one—the sun. Fresh air had been adopted as one of the weapons against tuberculosis in the United States because many immigrants who developed tuberculosis lived in crowded tenements and labored in factories without adequate ventilation. Social reform that could have slowed the spread of TB through better housing and working conditions faced a tough battle. Instead, fresh-air camps and sanatoriums embraced the open-air model—it was easy and cheap. Unfortunately, because pulmonary tuberculosis thrives in an oxygen-rich environment, the fresh-air-treatment that was presumed to be a cure could work against one by encouraging deep breathing and an influx of oxygen—the very fuel needed by the bacilli.

By 1921, information books for patients disparaged the belief that open air was necessary for treatment of tuberculosis.[1] Instead, they praised sunshine. In 1903, Dr. Niels Finsen of Denmark had received the Nobel Prize in Medicine for his work in using ultraviolet light to treat patients with tuberculosis of the skin. In the same year, Dr. Auguste Rollier initiated the use of sunbaths at his tuberculosis sanatorium in Leysin, Switzerland. By 1916, this treatment known as heliotherapy had become popular in America. Glen Lake's new infirmary featured many large windows for ventilation, but the ample porches were designed for sunbathing, not for air baths.

At the time, doctors were not entirely sure how the sun worked its benefits. Some believed the tanned skin had the ability to convert short ultraviolet rays into long ones.[2] Others assumed it worked by quickening circulation near the skin and triggering a chemical process that could kill the tuberculosis bacillus in the blood.[3] In 2010, more than 100 years after Rollier's adoption of heliotherapy, laboratory studies suggested that the link between the sun and tuberculosis is vitamin D. An increased supply of the vitamin may work by regulating the human body's supply of cathelicidin, an antimicrobial peptide that combats bacterial and viral infections, including *mycobacterium tuberculosis*.[4]

Heliotherapy did not work well for most pulmonary TB cases, however. Like fresh air, the sun could create a breeding ground, this time by raising a patient's temperature and increasing moisture in the lungs.[5]

In addition to helping patients with extra-pulmonary tuberculosis, heliotherapy was found to have a positive psychological effect, too. It gave patients an active role in their own cure, something tangible they could do besides lie in bed. Doctors found that patients keeping track of their "taking sun" time were amenable to much longer periods of bed rest. Heliotherapy helped ensure that people would stay in the sanatorium to receive maximum benefit from the most disagreeable component of treatment: confinement.[6]

Dr. Mariette embraced the concept of the sun cure and told the *Excelsior-Minnetonka Record* that, "Direct sunlight is the best germicide we have and we wanted as much as possible of it in the room, so we have tried to combine the room and the porch . . . each room is really only a glazed porch."[7] He recruited Dr. J. Harry Bendes from J.N. Adam Memorial Hospital in Perrysburg, New York, because it had been the first institution in the United States to employ a full-body approach to heliotherapy rather than localized exposure. Bendes quickly earned the nickname "sun doctor" from the patients.

The introduction of this method of heliotherapy to patients at Glen Lake produced surprisingly rapid and amazing results. A thirty-year-old woman had spent five years there, almost from the day the institution opened. A closed abscess on her spine and a painful open one on her left hip caused her leg to contract until her knee was over her abdomen. Treatment during her stay had consisted of confinement to a wooden bedframe with weights attached to her leg in hopes of straightening it. The severity of her pain made her indifferent to life. She was described as mentally only half alive and mercifully deadened.

When the new building unofficially opened in February, she and others with non-pulmonary tuberculosis were moved to the top floor, known as

Fifth Main, which was considered the "clean floor." All the patients had tuberculosis, but because it was not in the lung, no one had positive sputum.[8] Accommodations consisted of two ten-bed wards, one for women and one for men, and two double rooms for more acutely ill people.

The process was more complicated than merely putting the patient out in the sunlight. The regimen for exposure to the sun was carefully planned to encourage deep tans without burning the skin. The optimal time for treatment was early in the day, when the air was most free of dust and smoke and the sun's rays were not as hot on the skin. The first day, only the patient's feet were exposed to the sun, in four five-minute intervals. The next sunny day, her legs were exposed for that amount of time, and exposure to the feet was doubled. This process of gradually uncovering her entire body was continued until she received three hours of sun a day, in hour-and-a-half sessions. Her skin looked coppery at first, became bronzed, and ultimately took on a dark chocolate hue. More importantly, her pain was gone. She began to sleep better and regained an appetite. By April, the woman with non-pulmonary TB had been removed from the frame and the weights were gone. Her leg was straight and the abscesses were healing.[9]

She was not the only success story. More than twenty other patients were following the same regimen at the time, and all were becoming pain free and getting well. One peculiarity noted was that, contrary to expectations, the patients' deeply tanned skin was velvety and soft. The darkly

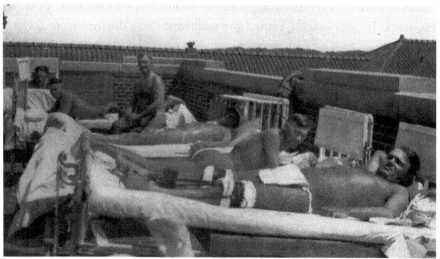

Heliotherapy—men sunbathing. (Courtesy of the Lokke Collection)

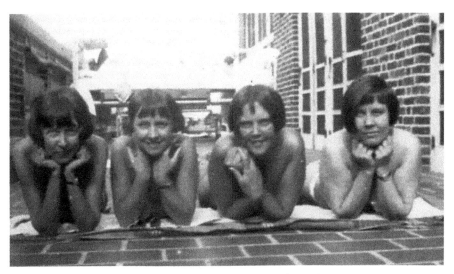

Heliotherapy—women sunbathing. (Courtesy of the Lokke Collection)

tanned skin did not pass without comment from the patients. Elizabeth Skagerberg, who may have contracted TB as a student nurse, placed an advertisement in the The *Arrow*'s "Wanted" section: "On fifth floor, my beautiful white skin." An unattributed poem submitted to the newsletter described how eagerly the "Suffering Sisters" and the gentlemen in Ward 511 watched for the sunrise.[10]

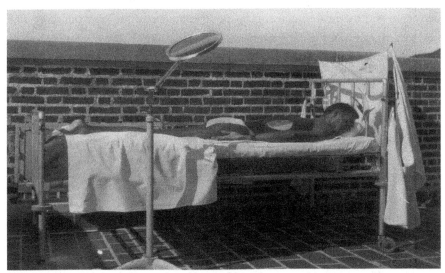

Man with Therzac Porsmeur lens. (Courtesy of the Hennepin History Museum)

In the case of patients who had skin lesions, a large lens called a Therzac Porsmeur lens would focus sunlight on particular areas. Individuals who did not tan easily were fed a diet rich in vitamins supplemented by cod liver oil. During Minnesota's coldest and least sunny winter months, the patients would lie under lamps that created artificial ultraviolet radiation.[11]

Lamp treatment was quite complicated, with differing types used at Glen Lake, including carbon arc, mercury quartz, and infra red. Carbon arc lamps were large and hung from the ceiling in a room used specifically for treatment of several patients at a time. The lamps provided a light that was the closest to natural sunlight. They were hot and illuminated the entire room, so patients wore eye protection during treatment. Glen Lake had one large carbon arc lamp in the infirmary building.

Mercury quartz and alpine floor lamps were used for individual treatments and had large aluminum hoods. The mercury quartz lamps did not provide as many red rays from the ultraviolet spectrum as did the carbon arc and alpine. They were considered to be less effective for general body treatment. The mercury quartz had stronger germicidal properties, but there was also more risk of irritating skin burns. Glen Lake had a portable water-cooled mercury lamp from the Hanovia Company for patients who required localized treatments. It could be adapted with applicators for specific lesions in the sinuses, throat, larynx, ears, nose, or skin areas.[12]

Dr. Mariette ensured that several other improvements and advances in patient care and medical practice were incorporated into the new building. The sanatorium's first X-ray equipment was installed. The X-ray, invented in 1895 by Wilhelm Roentgen, revealed shadows or cavities in the chests of otherwise healthy people. It helped physicians determine whether people who reacted to tuberculin tests had active tuberculosis. X-rays could also reveal scarring or hardening in the lungs, which indicated the TB was contained. The open bowls that held the X-ray tubes in the sanatorium's first machine probably drenched both the patient and the operator with unwanted radiation. "Bare wires carrying over a hundred thousand volts of he-man electricity offered possible death to him who came within a flea jump, but it was a means of getting the inside dope on ailing lungs," recalled one of the technicians.[13]

The new building also housed an official post office. In 1921, the U.S. Postal Service began direct service to the institution instead of through Hopkins. The name Hennco (for Hennepin County) had been proposed for the community's post office, but some of the women objected because the name sounded too much like hen coop. A contest was held among the patients, and the post office opened officially with Martha Barnett's winning name of Oak Terrace. Dr. Mariette served as postmaster, with former patient Oletta Desmond as the assistant postmaster.

Patients paid two cents to affix a first-class stamp to their letters home. Incoming and outgoing mail was dispatched on the fly from the trains that passed to the east of the sanatorium. Incoming mail was thrown from the train in sturdy bags; outgoing mailbags were retrieved by the train's catcher arm from a mail crane by the side of the track. This method was used because the train wasn't scheduled to stop at that crossing.[14] Within five years of becoming a post office, Oak Terrace handled more than 250 bags of mail per year.

As the sanatorium grew, so did its waiting list. In 1921, the list numbered 118 and included a father with tuberculosis. He was unemployed, infecting his family of six children, and developing into an advanced case. "Unless he can be given sanatorium care very shortly, he will pass the stage where a cure is possible," said an article in the *Minneapolis Morning Tribune*.[15]

So, even before the mortar was dry on the new infirmary, the Hennepin County commissioners and the Board of Public Welfare drafted a request to the Minnesota Legislature for more beds at the sanatorium. The $1,500,000 three-year bonding bill was approved. It provided for construction of a wing on each end of the infirmary, along with other structures on campus. Carl Wilwerding, president of the sanatorium's Trudeau Club, handed a pen to Governor Jacob Preus, and he signed the bill. The newly formed club, named after Dr. Edward Trudeau, counted all patients as members and planned social events for them. The daily newspaper reported that Wilwerding was on the "high road" to recovery and would soon leave the sanatorium.[16]

There had also been an ongoing effort for a facility in Hennepin County to care for children with tuberculosis. It had its genesis years earlier when various associations began to support fresh-air or summer camps for children. The camps were intended to build up resistance in children who were considered at risk for developing active tuberculosis.

Childhood tuberculosis could be in the lungs, as it was most commonly in adults, but it manifested primarily as a lymphatic disease. Tuberculosis meningitis was one of the most dreaded childhood diseases in early Minnesota. It would affect the central nervous system, usually near the base of the brain, and was invariably fatal.[17] Tuberculosis of the bone also created a serious situation for children. Without early treatment, they could spend the rest of their lives crippled, assuming they survived.[18]

Children who consumed unpasteurized milk from infected herds were at special risk because the bacilli entered the stomach and tended to migrate to organs and growing bones. An illustrated book of health jingles exhorted children to "learn every rhyme and be healthy all the time." One of the poems in *Muddy Jim and Other Rhymes* described how the gentle cow could be a menace:

When milk is raw just from the farm, It's full of germs which may do harm.
But safe it is and highly prized, When it is boiled or pasteurized.
Ice cream, cheese, and butter fat, Come from milk, you all know that.
Made from raw milk we can see, They might harm both you and me.[19]

The Minneapolis school district had already established open-air schools for children with tuberculous tendencies. A school supported by the Associated Charities' Anti-Tuberculosis Committee was set up in 1911 in a two-story building at Third Avenue and Eleventh Street. A second open-air school was opened in the Peabody building near Seven Corners. Both functions were eventually consolidated at Fourth Street and Ninth Avenue in the Thomas Arnold School, later renamed the Trudeau School. The pupils received four meals a day and studied with the windows open, even on the coldest days.[20]

While the Trudeau School educated children who were "pre-tuberculous," Lymanhurst Hospital School was founded in 1921 to educate and care for children with incipient tuberculosis. The property for the school at Chicago Avenue and Eighteenth Street was donated by two brothers, Fred and George Lyman. Associated with Minneapolis General Hospital but a block away from it, the school was equipped to diagnose and correct unrelated conditions, such as dental infections and congenital syphilis, which could hinder a return to good health.[21]

Because isolation was still seen as critical to stopping the spread of the disease, some cities built preventoriums, which were modeled after sanatoriums. They were built specifically to care for children who had been exposed to tuberculosis in their home, but who did not have active tuberculosis. Those children were deemed to be at particular risk of developing the disease because of malnutrition or other reasons, and a preventorium's function was to build up their resistance to the disease. The youngsters often came from poor or immigrant families, and a preventorium could function as an orphanage, with children living there for months or years.[22]

Ramsey County opened a Children's Preventorium in 1915, on the site of the former Cuenca Tuberculosis Sanatorium and Hospital on Bass Lake (now Lake Owasso in Shoreview), but Hennepin County did not have one at that time.[23] In 1916, J.R. Kingman, of the Hennepin County Sanatorium Commission, was appointed chairman of the Anti-Tuberculosis Committee, and he stated his intention to "use the funds and energies which have in the past built up the Open-Air school to obtain a preventorium for children at Glen Lake."[24]

The Christian family joined in his preventorium campaign, but unfortunately, Mrs. Christian died in 1916, at age seventy-one, before their goal could be achieved. Her husband died two years later, at the age of seventy-nine, also without seeing a children's building materialize at Glen Lake. His will left a million dollars to the Citizen's Aid Society, which took up their cause.[25] The Anti-Tuberculosis Committee supported this effort by passing a formal recommendation in 1918 that a preventorium for children should be erected on the grounds of the sanatorium.[26]

Nothing of substance happened, however, and in 1920, Kathryne Radebaugh noted the Thomas Arnold School was filled to capacity at ninety-six students, with a large waiting list. She also noted that few resources existed anywhere in the county for children who had active tuberculosis.[27]

By 1922, Glen Lake finally had its Children's Building, built with a $160,000 donation from the Citizen's Aid Society in memory of Lenore Christian. Furnishings were purchased from the proceeds of Christmas Seal sales, and the landscape gardening was contributed by H.E. Partridge. The Scottish Rite Women's Club of Minneapolis supplied clothing for the children.[28]

More than just a preventorium, it was equipped to provide three levels of care:

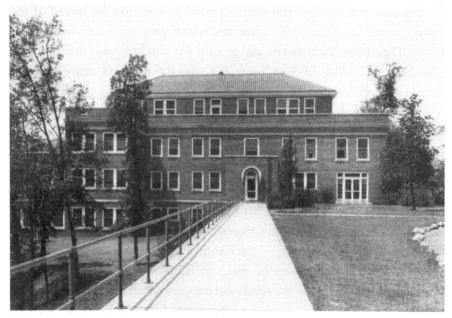

Children's building. (Courtesy of the Lokke Collection)

(1) building up of children who were predisposed to development of tuberculosis or exposed in the home,
(2) treating children afflicted with active tuberculosis, and
(3) caring for babies born of tuberculous mothers.[29]

The four-story building matched the main administration structure, being fire-resistant with a reinforced concrete and brick construction. It, too, was located on a slope of the main hill but stood to the west of and apart from the rest of the campus. The foundation level was exposed on the south side and held a big, airy playroom and a school room. The first floor had a reception room, the supervising nurse's office, a kitchen, two wards of twelve beds each, and a dining room, equipped with cheery child-sized furniture painted yellow with blue trim.

One end of the second floor held an apartment for five nurses. At the other end were two wards of twelve beds each, opening out onto balconies where the children would have heliotherapy on sunny days. Just as in the main building, an alpine lamp room could treat tuberculosis of the bone on sunless days.

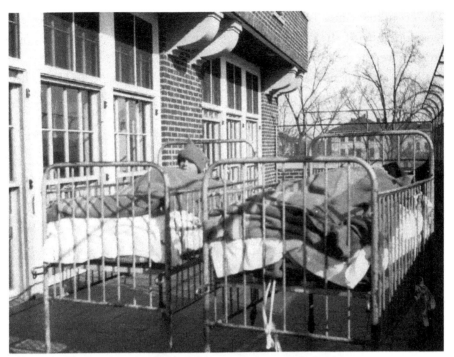

Children's heliotherapy. (Courtesy of the Minnesota Historical Society)

With all of the new construction, the Glen Lake campus expanded to 160 acres in 1924. The two wings were completed, with the east wing for men and the west for women. The mingling of sexes was strictly controlled, and the ability to segregate by location aided in enforcement of the rules. The wings were one story shorter than the main building, thus making the fourth floor the top level. Both Four East and Four West had large ten-bed wards on the south end of the wings, with floor-to-ceiling windows that allowed access to open porches. Patients on these floors needed sunbaths, but had other active tuberculosis that prevented them from being housed on the fifth floor of Main.

The east wing's basement housed a fully equipped morgue and laboratory facilities. The west wing's basement contained dormitory-style rooms used as lodging for female maids and dietary workers. The accommodations for staff were deemed necessary because of the distance from population centers and the streetcar station, the lack of individually owned cars, and the continuing stigma of having tuberculosis or working with people who did.

The economic status of employees at Glen Lake was reflected in the segregated nature of the campus housing. The lowest-earning employees quite literally lived in the lowest levels of the building.

New construction also included housing for nurses and female office employees in a building commonly known as the Nurses' Residence. It had

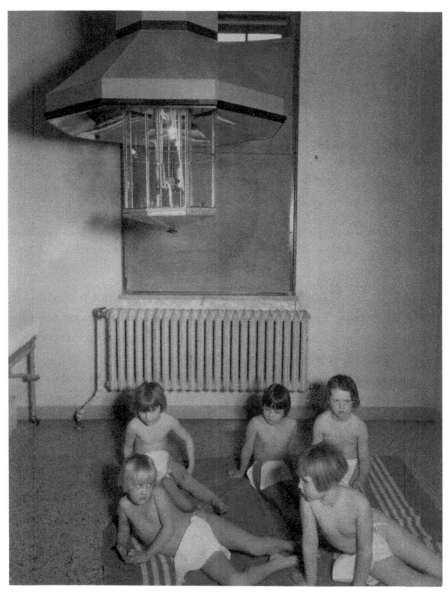

Alpine Lamp in the children's building. (Courtesy of the Hennepin History Museum)

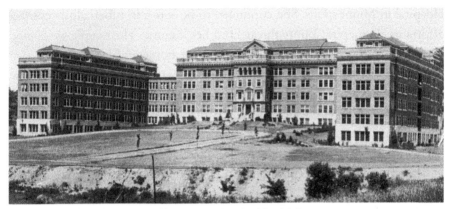

Wings completed. (Courtesy of the Hopkins Historical Society)

its own segregation, with nurses in one section and administrative staff, such as social workers and secretaries, in the other. Each woman had her own room, and there was maid service for bed-making and room cleaning. The large living room on the first floor was the only area in which men were allowed. It had a jukebox, a fireplace, and chairs and couches. The first floor also had a kitchen and a women-only living room.[30]

Homes for three physicians were built at a distance from the institution, on the north side of the campus. A physician's house was especially important to Dr. Mariette, who had married Anna Jones, niece of sanatorium commission member Edward Gale, in 1923. Before her marriage, she was an instructor in public health nursing and superintendent of nurses at Abbott

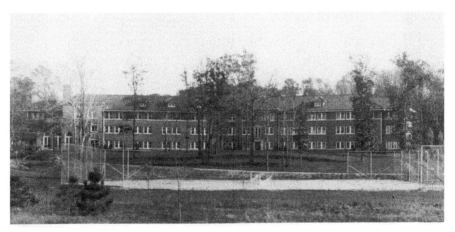

Nurses home. (Courtesy of the Hennepin History Museum)

Hospital in Minneapolis. She continued to be active in tuberculosis control efforts in Hennepin County throughout her lifetime. The couple welcomed Mariette's widowed mother, Grace, into their home and later adopted two children. Doctors Sumner Cohen and Peter Mattill and their families were long-term residents of the other two houses.

An auditorium connected the 1921 infirmary to the original 1916 administration building. A large, open archway between the main building and the auditorium allowed for ambulance access, but it meant that people either had to brave the elements to enter the auditorium or they had to go up to second floor to cross over and then return to the first floor. The design created a wind tunnel and patients dubbed the archway "Pneumo Alley." It was later enclosed.

In addition to the auditorium and the ambulance entrance, the connecting building contained the library, the Oak Terrace store for patients, several dining rooms, and an expanded kitchen with bakery. The upper floors of the connecting building provided bedrooms for kitchen staff.

An employee's building for men and married couples was built across the road to the south of the main campus. The accommodations in the employees' building included a caretaker couple who cleaned the individual rooms as well as the common spaces. The cleaning services served as a perk to lure employees to the sanatorium and was an important factor in the attempt to lessen the spread of all illnesses, including tuberculosis. Fresh towels were provided twice a week, and soap was free. The apartments were known as "Septic Heights" because of the proximity to the sewage settling tanks.[31]

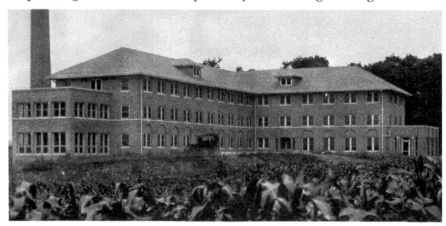

Men's building. (Courtesy of the Lokke Collection)

Next to the employee's building stood a new power plant that had capacity to serve the larger campus. A well, drilled 170 feet deep, provided nearly 25,000 gallons to the buildings each day for drinking, bathing, and cooking. A water-softening system added dehydrated lime to settling tanks, and the resulting water was sand-filtered before being pumped into a storage tank set into the hill behind the original sanatorium cottages.

The sanatorium also had its own waste-treatment system. Sewage came from the buildings through an underground line to a disposal tank behind

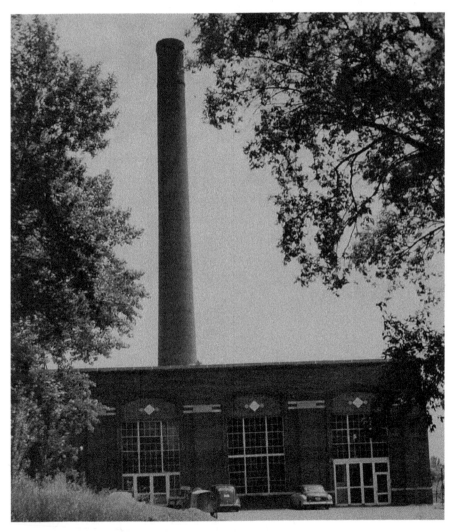

Power plant smokestack. (Courtesy of the Minnesota Historical Society)

the power house. After the sewage was de-aerated and treated with chlorine, the sludge was pumped into drying beds on the grounds. The water, when it left the sewage plant, was determined by the standards of the time to be of good quality and was discharged into the swamp area between the power house and Birch Island Lake. Patients knew the body of water by other names, including Sputum Lake and Enema Bay.[32]

Coal was delivered five or six railroad carloads at a time and was hand-shoveled into boilers that produced steam. The live steam drove generator units that made the electricity required by the institution. The steam also flowed into the heating system in the winter, went through the half-mile long tunnel to the main building, and circulated through radiators. During the summer, the steam was used to power the ice-making machine.

The power house's red brick smokestack towered above the trees and served as a neighborhood directional aid as well as the location of the steam whistle that signaled rest hours and visiting hours.

Even while Glen Lake expanded, the value of sanatorium care continued to be debated by both medical experts and community activists. Opponents cited high sanatorium-morbidity statistics and a preference for home care. Proponents pointed out that sanatorium death rates were high because patients admitted were often in advanced stages of the disease, and they argued for the community benefit of isolation.

6

Rest and Privileges

To COUNTERACT THE CRITICISM OF SANATORIUMS, Dr. Pottenger, in California, continued to advocate for patient isolation and easy access to a physician as the best means of defense against death.

> Should a patient go to a sanatorium? By all means, if he can. There is no other place where patients can get so good an idea of the disease, tuberculosis, as in a well-conducted sanatorium; no place where conditions are so favorable to cure; and no place where they will learn so well how to live the life necessary to retain health when once regained. . . . The moral support of others who have the same aim, who are living the same life and who are making the same sacrifices, is a tremendous factor in cure.[1]

Dr. Mariette strongly agreed with Dr. Pottenger's opinion of sanatoriums. By 1920, it was apparent that people could be healed of tuberculosis by allowing nature to do its work while lessening the efforts of the diseased lung. Because the lung moves up and down with breathing, it seemed logical to conclude that lying quietly in bed would encourage successful formation of the fibers needed to contain the germs. In the early stages of healing, the fibrous material laid down around the germs is extremely fine and web-like. It has little strength or consistency and is easily dislodged. Without disturbance, it can become progressively stronger and finally form a tough wall enclosing the tubercle bacilli. Complete bed rest was believed to also inhibit the spread of the tubercle bacilli to other parts of the body.[2]

Dr. Mariette clearly believed that the new regimen of bed rest was essential to recovery. He told potential patients, "Everything worth owning costs something; to regain your health will cost something; the price will be the strict adherence to routine and rules of the sanatorium. Is your health worth it? If not, this is not the place for you."[3]

A series of events called "privileges" became the milestones for each patient's road to home, and this method of classification continued into the 1950s. The system was well defined and recorded in a desk book located in the sanatorium's reception area. Incoming patients were given a handbook that explained the routine and rules. Each patient had differing needs, of course, but physicians who were considering deviations from procedures were expected to present their reasons at the weekly medical staff meetings. The group would discuss the patient's situation and make recommendations for exceptions.[4]

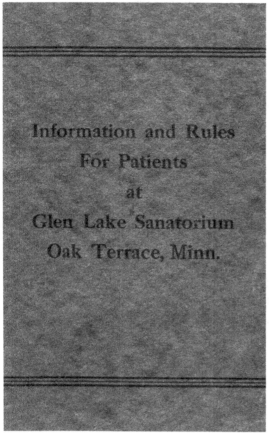

Glen Lake Sanatorium Handbook. (Author's collection)

All stays at Glen Lake Sanatorium started with intensive bed rest, which meant having patients lie completely flat to achieve maximum idleness. The patients could read or feed themselves only with their physician's permission. This observation period lasted about six weeks because intake examinations and tests took that long.

The next step was strict bed, which could stretch to six months or longer. If only one lung was affected, the patient might be instructed to do postural rest. That required lying on the diseased side for at least twenty-three hours a day, with sandbags fore and aft to further inhibit breathing with that lung.[5]

58

When not required to do postural rest, patients still had to lie in bed, but could have limited activity, such as writing letters and feeding themselves. They could leave their rooms on litters (wheeled cots) once every two weeks, with their physician's permission, to attend church or an entertainment.[6]

Patients did not wear hospital gowns, but were not allowed to wear "street" clothes, either. Most wore pajamas and robes.[7] Beatrice Olson had a special pair of pink satin pajamas with a matching pink afghan that she would wear to church and shows.[8] Women who were not on strict bed were

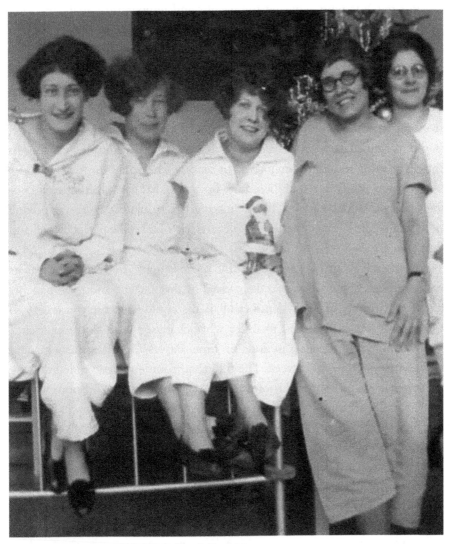

Typical apparel. (Courtesy of the Lokke Collection)

allowed to wear blouses instead of a pajama top. There was a standard joke that greeted a person who finally was up and dressed in normal clothing: "Well, I didn't know you with your clothes on."[9]

Patients at Glen Lake knew the two goals they needed to attain to move forward in the privilege system: weight gain and a normal body temperature. Most patients took and recorded their own temperature each morning and, until 1940, it was with a rectal thermometer because the doctors believed that was more accurate.[10]

For patients who achieved the weight and temperature goals, the next step after strict bed was regular bed, which allowed them to be propped up to eat, read, or do craftwork. They could also ride in a wheelchair instead of on a litter for the trips to the auditorium or treatments, and they could attend one social activity a week.

The very first privilege, one bathroom, gave patients a limited escape from their bed. It allowed one trip to the bathroom each day (preferably for a bowel movement). They also gained permission to walk from the elevator to the chairs into the auditorium instead of using a wheelchair for the entire trip.

Howard Johnson remembered the first time that he walked after spending a year on strict bed rest: "The railing was pretty handy. My legs just didn't hold me. While I was in bed I did no exercises. I had to lie perfectly still and flat. I wasn't allowed to sit up."[11]

With each bathroom privilege came more activity. Two bathroom, as its name implies, allowed for two daily visits to that facility, and male patients could shave there instead of in bed. Patients could walk the whole way to the auditorium, but needed to use a wheelchair for visits and treatments, to avoid standing for long periods of time. Passes for entertainments and church increased to two a week. The three bathroom privilege added walking to treatments, and four bathroom was just that—an extra bathroom visit.

The full bathroom privilege meant taking a tub bath or shower. That was a real treat for patients after months or even years of bed baths.

The semi-ambulant privilege allowed the patient to go to the dining room for a meal. This started with one trip to the dining room. First-timer men went to the dining room at noon; women to the evening meal.

Once a patient had graduated to eating all three meals in the dining room, they were considered ambulant. They enjoyed a half hour of exercise, which could be taken as an outdoor walk in the evening during warm weather. As the exercise was increased they started doing odd jobs as part of a routine of working up to going home. Some people delivered newspapers, picked up magazines, or ran the elevators. They didn't get paid for it; it was part of testing their recovery and preparing them for discharge.[12]

Ambulant patients were also eligible for leaves, which could range from eight or ten hours to a few days. Frances Melby, who lived on a farm near Montevideo, Minnesota, remembered her cousin Ruby Botten coming from Glen Lake to visit them occasionally for a weekend. After each meal, though, Frances's mother would boil all of the dishes.[13]

Although the leaves were not based on good behavior, a patient's "bad" behavior could result in the cancellation of a leave. Bad behavior could include smoking in the buildings, fraternizing with the opposite sex, or not being in bed by lights out. Those were the rules that rankled patients the most. Even fifty-year-olds were made to feel like they were sixteen again, subjected to parental discipline.

Most requests for leaves of absence were for seasonal and religious holidays. The medical staff decided that Jewish patients who wished to celebrate the Jewish holidays could receive leaves to do so if their condition permitted, but they were not to also request leaves on the Gentile holidays.[14]

As patients continued to improve and their tuberculosis was contained, the last step was moving to the cottages, to semi-private rooms for men in the East Cottage and the same for women in the West Cottage. The tunnel system connected to the main building's facilities, so patients didn't have to go outside during the winter. While there was always a nurse on duty to dispense medications and handle emergencies, this halfway-house setup helped transition the patients from dependency to taking care of themselves. Along with working in the institution, they were allowed to come and go pretty much as they pleased until curfew.[15] Four hours was selected as the maximum exercise because it was felt that if the patient could stand four hours of exercise without reactivating his disease, he would have an excellent chance of remaining well after leaving the sanatorium.[16]

Speculation on when privileges would begin was a frequent topic of conversation. It was worthy of publication in the sanatorium magazine when the event finally happened, as in this note: "Congratulations are in order for Nancy S., Fifth Adm., who after exactly one year in bed received her first privilege on Memorial Day."[17]

Esther Giere Johnson wrote in her diary: "When Dr. Fenger made rounds today he gave me a PRIVILEGE [emphasis in original]."[18]

Rarely, though, did patients progress straight through all levels without a relapse sending them back to a previous level, like a cruel game of Chutes and Ladders.

Maryanna Shorba's diary described the granting of a privilege in January: "Greatest joy that I'm getting up! And shock almost too much. Now if I stay there. Glad adhesion is okay and my trouble practically healed." Three weeks later, she noted a "Crazy stitch in side. What's that now?" She lost the privilege and was wistful: "Wish had privilege." As she experienced several better-and-worse cycles, she expressed anger: "Yes, goddamn stuff's probably returning," and despair: "Chest feels awful. Just wonder where I'll come out. God, be with me." It would be September before she finally attained three bathroom and began working up to the West Cottage and her discharge in June of the next year, one and a half years after her first privilege.[19]

The rigidity of the privilege system was matched by the military-like regimentation of the daily schedule. Frederick Manfred wrote in a letter to a friend, "The day starts for us at seven when the sputum cup collector comes into the room with a tray and a barely suppressed flashlight. A few minutes later nurses barge in."[20] The remainder of the day followed the schedule:

7:30 a.m.	Breakfast, followed by bed-making, shaving, and other personal care.
9:00 a.m.	From 9 until 11:15, either rest or exercise, as prescribed by a doctor.
10:00 a.m.	Morning lunch for underweight patients.
11:15–11:45 a.m.	Rest period—complete, with no exercise, talking, reading, or knitting. All patients were expected to be in bed.
11:45 a.m.	Social half hour in the lobby for patients of both genders who were ambulant or semi-ambulant.
12:15 p.m.	Noon dinner.
1:00 p.m.	Rest period for all patients, with sleeping expected. Nursing staff was also encouraged to rest.
3:00 p.m.	Two hours allowed for rest or exercise as prescribed.
3:30 p.m.	Lunch for underweight patients.
5:00 p.m.	Social half hour.
5:30 p.m.	Supper.

6:00–7:00 p.m.	Rest hour with patients in bed and lights out. A radio concert was broadcast at this time.
7:00 p.m.	Recreation hour, especially for ambulent and semi-ambulant patients, who could gather in the auditorium or movie nights on Wednesdays.
8:00 p.m.	Evening lunch for underweight patients.
9:00 p.m.	Lights out.

Restricting personal freedom for such extreme lengths of time was possible in an era when people were accustomed to a physician's authority and would follow the structure of medical care. Doctors were assumed to know best, and patients were expected to obey without questioning. Still, the disciplined regulation of the sanatorium took precedence over individual rights in a way that often annoyed the patients confined to bed.[21]

Dr. Pottenger, in his book for patients, described this period of enforced rest as an opportunity for a patient to develop new habits of survival: "The person who cannot face the circumstances forced upon him by his disease, and develop habits compatible with his new mode of living, is not going to get along as well as his roommate with the same extent of disease who can make the adjustment." He said a patient who would not "program" was an unsatisfactory patient and a bad influence on other patients with whom he came in contact. "He is the one who gives physicians troubles in a sanatorium. He will not obey rules and he prevents others from doing so," he wrote. He also said that the patient who disliked this program and discipline the most was, as a rule, the one who needed it most.[22]

Sadie Fuller Seagrave, who was a patient at Ah-gwah-ching Sanatorium at Walker, Minnesota, published a memoir in 1918. She thought the personal quality that helped her most to win the fight against tuberculosis was patience: patience with rigid discipline, patience with other patients, and patience with the length of time necessary to heal.[23]

All of the patients, whether strict bed or not, were expected to comply with rest hours. So was nearly everyone who worked at the sanatorium. The steam whistle on the smokestack of the power plant signaled the beginning and end of rest hours three times a day.[24]

It might seem superfluous to require specific rest hours for people confined to bed, but Dr. Mariette said that rest periods were necessary for patients because of the mental activity of observing people around them.[25]

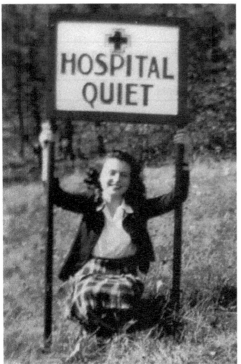

Quiet sign. (Courtesy of Lanners Collection)

Esther Giere Johnson noticed the difference when she moved from Three West (a quiet intensive-care floor) to Four West. She wrote in her diary, "Became very tired by the extra noises and confusion at first, but I'm getting used to it."[26]

The sanatorium was a fairly noisy place. Marble, brick, concrete, and plaster reflected sound. For the sake of cleanliness, the building lacked homey touches such as wallpaper, pictures, and curtains, which might have absorbed noise. The beds were metal, as were the bedside tables. Meals were served on heavy china dishes with metal utensils. Liquids were served in glass or aluminum containers. Bedpans were enameled metal. The windows were wood-framed and double or triple hung. They shrank and rattled from the winter's dryness and swelled and stuck in summer's humidity.

The afternoon rest hour, especially, was intended to be as quiet as possible. Window shades were pulled down, and there was no coming or going. Patients couldn't read or do craftwork. The daytime nursing staff worked split shifts to accommodate the afternoon rest period, coming to work at 7:00 a.m. and being off duty from 12:30 p.m. until 3:00 p.m. They then came back to do the afternoon cares and serve supper before being relieved by the evening shift.[27]

This pattern of limited activity balanced with rest continued throughout the sanatorium era, and so did the complaints about the semi-incarceration. Dr. William Carroll responded to complainers, "The program which is adopted by those who treat tuberculosis is based on study and experience. It is not adopted for fun or for punishment of patients."[28]

Manfred had a roommate who he was sure would survive tuberculosis, because the young man was always complaining. He hated being there, and he was full of endless questions. Manfred thought, "Well, that's pretty good, he's probably going to live, he's got life in him, he wants to fight to stay alive . . . I figured I'd never make it. I didn't have that fire." The roommate, who resisted rules and fought to live, didn't survive. Manfred speculated that perhaps he himself lived because he followed the rules like he was told to.[29]

Regardless of the perceived benefits of bed rest and a sanatorium stay, there was no avoiding the reality of an extended disruption of normal life. Researchers Geoffrey Bowker and Susan Star have noted, "Not knowing how long one will be incarcerated, not having any milestones or turning points that make sense, also makes time seem endless . . ."[30]

Julius Roth, author of a sociological study, said that a TB patient regarded his treatment "largely in terms of putting in time rather than in terms of the changes that occur in his lungs." This perception would lead to each patient "frantically trying to find out how long he is in for."[31]

Before a cure was discovered, patients could be at a sanatorium for a long time. Indeed, the Minnesota Legislature did not limit the length of time a patient could remain in a county sanatorium, leading to years-long treatments. Dr. Mariette even thought that the effectiveness of the sanatorium treatment could be measured by the length of stay because patients had time to learn how to live more healthfully before rejoining their families and the community.[32] He emphasized that hospitalization should always be considered indefinite and depended solely on an individual's response to treatment.[33]

New patients responded to this ambiguity by pestering the physicians and nurses. When Manfred marveled at a previous resident's sixteen-year recovery and asked, "Do I have to stay here that long?" it was a question no one could answer.

Doctors wished they could answer it, though, and developed various classification systems that would give them benchmarks for gauging a patient's capacity to resume a normal life outside of the sanatorium. They knew the final standard set by the National Tuberculosis Association, which was that discharge should be based on a diagnosis of either "arrested" or "quiescent." Both called for all constitutional symptoms to be absent. Sputum, if any, had to be negative for tubercle bacilli, with X-ray findings showing a stationary or retrogressive lesion. For arrested, these conditions needed to have existed for six months, during the last two of which the patient had been taking one hour's exercise. A finding of quiescent allowed for the same conditions existing for two months.

Systems of benchmarks differed among institutions. Common ones were based on the alphabet or numbers, which might also be accompanied by bed assignment according to designated wards or floors. Those classification systems could create discontent by leading patients to believe, erroneously, that they could judge the nearness of discharge based on assignments. Roth quoted a patient in his study as saying, "It's like an ungraded schoolroom."[34]

For the first years of Glen Lake's existence, only the patients taking sun cures outdoors were actively participating in any treatment that offered hope of a cure. Pulmonary TB patients on bed rest could participate only by doing nothing. Their temperature readings and weight gains could fluctuate wildly, without any apparent involvement from them, either negative or positive.

Many patients at Glen Lake had little to do except keep track of time's passing, somewhat like cartoon prisoners carving slashes on their cell walls. One woman obtained safety pins from the laundry and displayed a pin for every week she lived at the sanatorium.[35] Calendars were popular ways to mark the days, as were diaries, such as those kept by Maryanna Shorba, Esther Giere Johnson, and Hannah Lokke.

While the patients kept track of time, Dr. Mariette kept the sanatorium up to date on the latest medical treatments. Rest and heliotherapy continued to be the primary prescriptions, but they were increasingly augmented with surgical interventions. Although the medical procedures by themselves presented yet another passive role for patients, they, nevertheless, offered increased involvement in decisions about treatment. The era of complete and passive bed rest was slowly passing, and sanatoriums like Glen Lake embraced the advances that modern medicine offered.

January 18   Tuesday -

Dr. Funk and Dr. Satherlie (our new Interne) made rounds in a.m. No one in here got a speck of mail all day today - Selma came out to see me in evening - Miss Foreman was our night nurse. I sneaked in 246 and visited with the girls after Selma left. 7 a.m. 98⁶ - 70 - 0 = 3 p.m. 98⁸ 70 - 1 = 7 p.m. 99² - 74 - Gene Tunney was here during rest hour so we did not see him -

January 19   Wednesday.

Dr. Satherlie made rounds in a.m. - I got a letter from Nellie O'Neil, and Petra Kjeldsgard - I sneaked in 254 in evening to see Helen. Charles Lovequen was our orderlie today as Mike has today off. 7 a.m. 98° - 68 - 0 = 3 p.m. 98⁸ 70 - 1 = 7 p.m. 99² - 78 - Miss Foreman is our night nurse.

January 20 -   Thursday -

I got a letter from John and one from Nora Brown our (ministers son) Ed Ferris was in to see us this P.M. he did not know any ones name in here so he had quite a job getting a pass as he happened to think Julia started with "Malm" so he told them and they looked up a "Malm (something) in 242 and found out it was Malmberg so he got a pass for her. Miss Foreman was our night nurse - 7 a.m. 98⁴ - 68 - 0 = 3 p.m. 98⁶ - 72 - 1 = 7 p.m. 99 - 72.

Diary page. (Courtesy of the Lokke Collection)

7

Surgery

As SURGICAL INTERVENTIONS BECAME more common at the sanatorium, patients and their families could participate in discussions about the surgery. They were able to refuse if they so wished. Most patients chose to have operations performed at Glen Lake, but they could opt to go to a hospital where a consultant would be the primary surgeon. Even recovery

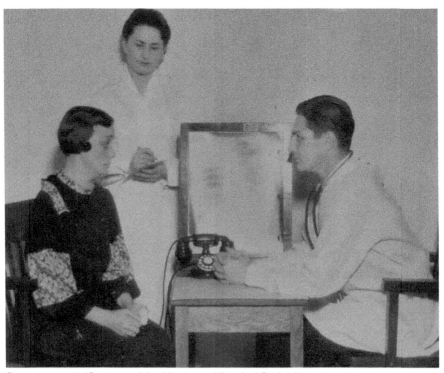

Surgery consult. (Courtesy of the Minnesota Historical Society)

from surgery offered more opportunity for, or at least the illusion of, greater participation in the healing process.

The first procedure to be introduced at Glen Lake was called pneumothorax (air plus chest). Doctors in England had noticed as early as 1835 that a spontaneous collapse of a lung was sometimes followed by improvement in a tuberculous patient's health. In our lungs, there are two layers of pleura: one is the covering for the lung, and the other lines the chest cavity. These pleural surfaces are entirely separate from each other but are in close contact. When these pleural surfaces are separated from each other by air, the lung can be collapsed. With the lung pushed into a state of inactivity, the body can more efficiently perform its task of encapsulating the tuberculosis bacilli.[1]

In the 1880s, an Italian physician, Carlo Forlanini, successfully inserted air via a needle and produced an artificial pneumothorax. The procedure was recommended at the annual meeting of the American Medical Association in 1889, and Minnesota's Dr. Henry Longstreet Taylor treated a patient by artificial pneumothorax in 1899, but it was not often employed. Artificial pneumothorax did not become popular in America until doctors serving in

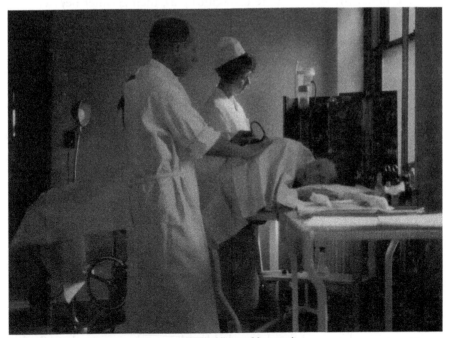

Pneumotherapy. (Courtesy of the Hennepin History Museum)

Europe during World War I learned that it had become a standard form of therapy for tuberculosis in several countries.[2]

To establish a pneumothorax, from 150 to 300 cubic centimeters of air would be inserted via needle every day or every other day until the lung achieved the desired state of collapse. It needed to be done gradually because it was painful to have a needle inserted between the ribs, even with anesthesia, and it was unnerving to lose breathing capacity. As more of the lung was collapsed, it became less painful.[3]

Glen Lake entered this new phase of medical therapy when artificial pneumothorax was first performed there in 1922. One patient described "pneumo" from his point of view. After checking out material from the library and learning everything that could go wrong with the procedure (air embolisms, fungi growth) he found the actual procedure a bit anticlimactic.

> I lay still while the nurse painted a spot under my arm with iodine and then washed it off. The doctor showed me the pneumo machine, explained how the air passed through various solutions which cleansed and purified it . . . I felt the Novocain describe an arc under my skin. A knife came into play, then another needle. Out of the corner of my eye I saw a red tube being connected with the needle . . . "One hundred," said the nurse. I stiffened. I could sense impending disaster. "Two hundred," announced the nurse. "That's all," said the doctor. "A piece of tape, please." He stripped off his rubber gloves. It was over and I was on my way back to my room with chastened spirits. I felt let down.[4]

Because the air would be slowly absorbed by the tissues, the procedure needed to be repeated on a regular basis to maintain the collapse.[5] A negative pressure existed in the intra-pleural space between the two coverings, so the doctor would take "pneumo readings" to determine the negative pressure and decide how much air would be introduced at a refill. The average refill ranged from 300 to 500 cubic centimeters. The procedure reminded patients of inflating a tire.

A fluoroscope machine was used in conjunction with the procedure to allow the physician to determine sufficient collapse. The patient stood against the machine and the doctor held and moved a screen that allowed

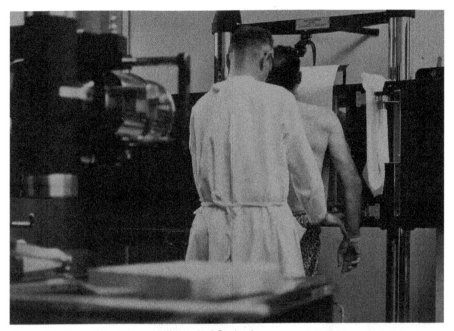

X-ray. (Courtesy of the Minnesota Historical Society)

him to see internal organs. The radiation from this procedure has since been found to have caused a higher rate of breast cancer in women who had this done multiple times.[6]

Some days as many as forty people would be in line waiting for the doctors to inject air.[7] If the procedure was successful, the injections of air might be discontinued within a year or two. Many people continued to "get air" for several years after discharge from the sanatorium.[8] Pneumothorax also benefitted the community indirectly. A collapsed lung was less likely to shed bacteria, which was important for decreasing contagion among people. Because it didn't involve extensive surgery, almost all sanatoriums administered pneumotherapy as part of routine treatment.

When a patient had an accidental leakage of air from the lung and experienced an unintended and unwanted spontaneous pneumothorax, the doctor would prescribe constant suction to re-expand the lung. In the summer, suction was created with an electric motor and pump. At Glen Lake in the winter it was uniquely and more quietly provided by the cast iron radiator in the patient's room. The sanatorium's mechanical engineer designed a "Vacuum Regulating Valve" and the workshop built it. The steam lines returning to

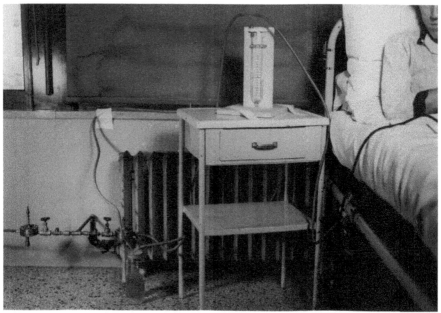

Suction machine. (Courtesy of the Hennepin History Museum)

the boilers at the power plant were used to produce suction on the lung. This had the advantage of being always constant, never interrupted.[9]

Sometimes the artificial pneumothorax procedure wasn't successful because the diseased part of the lung had already adhered to the cavity and wouldn't collapse. Other surgical interventions could be performed at the sanatorium because of the fully functional operating room in the Main building. Several methods all had the same aim: immobilization and collapse of the lung. For example, a phrenectomy cut or crushed the phrenic nerve on either the right or left side and paralyzed the diaphragm. That allowed it to retract into the thoracic cavity under the corresponding lung and limit its movement.[10]

Extrapleural thoracoplasty was another procedure that gained popularity in Europe almost twenty years before it became an accepted treatment in the United States. This surgery is permanent and irreversible because it is basically the removal of ribs, although the rib covering is allowed to remain. New rib bones will regenerate, but because they re-grow in the configuration of the already collapsed lung, the chest wall remains in a depressed position. The number and length of ribs removed was determined by what seemed necessary in each case. If more than three ribs needed to be removed, it was done in stages.[11]

The first thoracoplasty done in Minnesota was at the Mayo Clinic in 1919.[12] The first procedure at Glen Lake was done in 1922 by Dr. Arthur A. Law on a sixty-two-year-old patient. The second operation was on a twenty-four-year-old woman. The former lived to be eighty and the latter was reported as still healthy in 1949.[13]

Beatrice Olson, a patient at the sanatorium, had two stages of thoracoplasty and said it was quite painful afterwards. One stage did not collapse the cavity as hoped, so they did a second stage. While the procedure did not create a deformity for her, the operation could result in a droopy shoulder or concave chest.[14]

The removal of ribs, because it was done from the back, became known as a "spine hemstitching" among the patients.[15] It also gave rise to dark humor about rib removal, to the extent that the dietary department ceased serving pork or beef ribs at meals for a while. One patient organized the Mystic Order of the Short Rib, complete with a membership card signed by him as the Keeper of the Royal Bone Yard.[16]

Bronchoscopic examinations to detect or remove tuberculous lesions began at Glen Lake in 1926 by Dr. Kenneth Phelps. Tuberculosis of the trachea and bronchi was occasionally a complication in people who otherwise had a non-tuberculous pulmonary disease. With the bronchoscope, diseased tissue could be removed for laboratory study before employing more extensive surgical procedures.[17]

The aim of all interventions was to achieve a healing of the lungs. In the 1920s, methods for ascertaining the extent of healing were still limited. One of the critical measures of readiness for life outside the sanatorium included study of patients' sputum or stomach juices.

Mucus, called phlegm when produced in the lower air passages, is called sputum when expectorated by coughing or spitting. Sputum spreads the tuberculous bacilli and must be handled as contaminated waste. It could be argued that the major contribution of sanatoriums was, in fact, their role in preventing the spread of tuberculosis. Patients believed they should be discharged when they felt better, but doctors wanted them to stay until their sputum was no longer a source of danger and infection to others.

The patients' infectious sputum was also their own worst enemy. When swallowed, it could lead to the spread of tuberculosis because stomach acids do not kill the bacilli. It causes no problem in the stomach, but the lymphoid tissue in the intestine is easily infected, and that drains into the blood system, allowing dissemination throughout the body.[18]

For their own safety and that of others, patients were required to expectorate their sputum into a cup. Patients with active tuberculosis were required to have a sputum cup near them at all times. Ambulant patients carried wax-covered flat pocket cups with a flap. Johnson & Johnson made a Lister's Pocket Sputum Cup that was made of two layers of cardboard with a waterproof center.

The bedside sputum cup was a solid metal or wire container that contained a paper insert with flaps. When the inner cup was about one-half full, a nurse would remove the insert, fill it to the top with sawdust, fold in the flaps, and place it on a special shelf. The sawdust absorbed the sputum to prevent spills, and it also aided destruction of the cups by fire. An employee known as the cup man would collect the pocket cups and inserts and bring

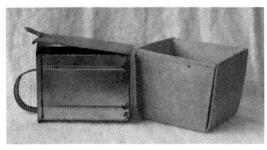

Sputum cup. (Author's collection)

them to the incinerator at the power house. He would also collect the dirty containers for sterilizing and deliver clean ones. The sanatorium patients used about 150,000 paper cups a year.[19]

To test sputum, the patient coughed into a sterile cup. The laboratory technician used a centrifuge to spin the sputum until bacilli were forced to the bottom, and then the residue was inoculated into a healthy guinea pig. The animals were used because it required about 100,000 tubercle bacilli per cubic centimeter of sputum in order to be seen through a microscope in a stained smear, but it took only a few tubercle bacilli to infect a guinea pig. The guinea pig was allowed to live for six weeks, and then it was killed and its organs were examined for the presence of tubercles. If proper precautions had been taken, the doctor could be sure that any tuberculosis found in the guinea pig came from the infected patient.[20]

About 700 guinea pigs were used at Glen Lake each year, costing from fifty to sixty cents apiece. Besides the actual cost of the guinea pigs, there was the expense of maintaining them. Most of them were raised in-house, and some were purchased from the University of Minnesota. Because the guinea pigs and their cages had an offensive odor, the lab was moved several times until finally settling into a permanent home in the power plant.

If bovine tuberculosis was suspected, a rabbit was used and it was inoculated through a vein in the ear. Chickens were used for the blood work of an avian type of tuberculosis, which was rare.[21]

The other test to endure was a gastric lavage, which retrieved stomach liquids for testing. The patient had two choices: swallow the lubricated rubber tubing or have it inserted via the nose. When the tubing entered the stomach, the technician would draw out the liquid needed, and then the tubing would be rapidly pulled out.[22]

A few patients decided not to have surgical treatment. They were asked to complete and sign a form in the presence of a witness, who also would sign it:

I have been advised by the Staff of Glen Lake Sanatorium to have a _____ but hereby refuse to follow this advice and assume full responsibility for anything which may develop as a result of this action.[23]

Some patients not only refused treatment, but refused to sign the form. Then the following had to be noted on a statement in the presence of the patient: "This patient not only refuses treatment but is uncooperative as well and refuses to sign this statement."[24]

In *Bargaining for Life*, Barbara Bates states, "the separation of sanatoriums from the mainstream of health care had left them uninformed and inexperienced."[25] This was not true of sanatoriums that reaped the benefit of being associated with a medical school or general hospital, thus having several consulting physicians available. Glen Lake's physical proximity to a major population center and several hospitals greatly increased the number and type of services it could offer. A report in 1926 named thirty-five consulting physicians, with specialties including dermatology, otolaryngology, pediatrics, gynecology, and urology.

In a span of just four years, from 1925 to 1929, the combination of medical care and surgery at Glen Lake had decreased the annual death rate of patients with far-advanced tuberculosis from eighty percent to fifty-seven-and-a-half percent.[26] That rate improved still more in the 1930s, when an addition to the building included modern surgical suites. The new facilities permitted more operations to be performed on-site and decreased the trauma resulting from transfers to other hospitals. Although the surgical interventions became popular at many sanatoriums, Mark Caldwell points out in his book, *The Last Crusade*, that thoracoplasty and pneumothorax were never scientifically proven to be effective in halting the spread of the disease. If the patient improved, perhaps the reason was the patient's own constitution.[27]

The surgeries continued at Glen Lake, however, with the lowering death rate used as justification. But, even with fewer patients dying, the specter of death still haunted patients every day. Averaging one or two deaths a week is significant in a community of 600 patients. All patients knew something about the other patients, even if only their name. Glen Lake, like most sanatoriums in the U.S., avoided mentioning death and discouraged talk of it by patients.

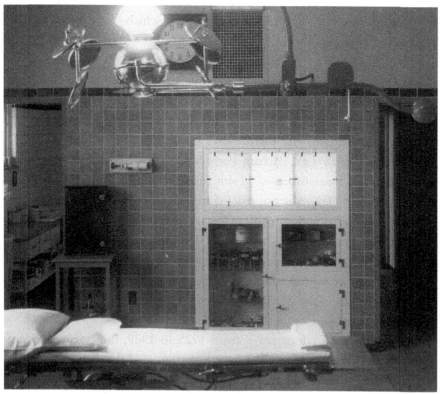

New operating room. (Courtesy of the Hennepin History Museum)

8

Death and Dying

THERE WERE NO OBVIOUS REPRESENTATIONS of death at Glen Lake. The sanatorium newsletter did not include death notices, and memorial services were not held at the sanatorium. Public expressions of grief were seen as negative experiences that could hinder recovery. American attitudes toward dying have changed since the publication of Elisabeth Kübler-Ross's book *On Death and Dying* in 1969, but in the sanatorium era, discussing death with a terminal patient was considered a cruel and uncaring thing to do.

When Sarah Weisman's children wanted to create a memorial to her at Glen Lake, it was the subject of much discussion. Her children wished to furnish and name a room in memory of their mother. An idea like this had never before been presented to the staff, and they worried about the effect a memorial might have on patients. After much arguing pro and con, Dr. Mariette and Miss Ridler approved the request and door 305 acquired a bronze plaque "In memory of Sarah Weisman."[1]

There are no references to death and dying in the handbooks given to new patients, but one would not expect the table of contents to have an entry for "death." Other publications written for sanatorium patients, usually by former patients, tended to be inspirational. Edward Hayes, a physician who took the "cure" and wrote a book about it, did not refer to death or dying. Instead, he discussed the "fear of not getting well" and having the right emotional attitude toward conquering illness.[2]

Other authors were more forthright about their fears. Will Ross, who spent five years in a sanatorium in Wisconsin in the early 1900s, wrote about his reaction to a thunderstorm. "It made me afraid; it made me think of death. It made me think of that vague eternity up back of the angry clouds that were pouring their heart on the earth. I wanted no part of it; I wanted to live."[3]

At Glen Lake, the emphasis was on "living with tuberculosis." Although discussion of death was discouraged, reminders of life's fragility were as close as the next bed. Beatrice Olson's roommate, a seventeen-year-old girl, said that she didn't mind dying, she just didn't want to die so young. Unfortunately, she couldn't undergo any of the usual medical interventions because the tuberculosis was too low in her lungs.[4]

Death from tuberculosis was not the gentle fading away depicted in movies. People in the end stages of pulmonary tuberculosis were likely to be coughing frequently, which disturbed their roommates both physically and emotionally. A fatal hemorrhage might occur. The eruption of blood from the mouth and the nose would be a disturbing event to witness. When Harold Faucher suffered a hemorrhage at home, his fiancée, Lucille Steinhagen, helped his mother re-wallpaper the bedroom. Harold was admitted to the Veterans' Hospital, but by the time he was discharged, Steinhagen was at Glen Lake fighting her own battle with TB.[5]

Extremely ill people were moved out of wards to single rooms or to the third floor intensive care units of the east and west wings.[6] These setbacks were mentioned indirectly in the newsletter with upbeat expressions. One typical entry reported that "Gerald S. has gone up for a quick overhaul." The "gone up" phrase and similar euphemisms meant that someone had suffered a serious relapse and was moved to the third floor. The First West gossip column reported that Dagne, Peggy, and Betty were all leaving for short visits to Third West and wished them the best of luck. One man's pals on Main East said, "We were all sorry to see Mr. B. leave for third floor and hoping he will be back on ME soon."[7]

In private, the move to third floor was expressed more honestly. "Poor Margaret had to move, so sick, will she ever be well?" was how Maryanna Shorba told her diary about a roommate's transfer to Third West.[8]

The state of one's health was a constant concern at the sanatorium. Esther Giere Johnson recorded her medical procedures in her diary, sometimes in great detail. "Had my cysto today. Lots of pain afterwards. They gave me a hypo. I had a blue pill before I went down, and a chill when I got on the table. . . . I developed a drastic emesis. Seemed like I'd turn inside out."[9] Esther's last entry was in August 1933, when she was discharged. She was readmitted, discharged, and readmitted again in 1934. She died at Glen Lake on June 23, 1936.

Every X-ray was an occasion to worry. If the spot on someone's lung spread, it was devastating news for everyone who knew them. People who seemed to be on the road to recovery would hemorrhage and die. Others would rally from the brink and live. Many had experienced already encountered death because of tuberculosis in their families. Frederick Manfred recalled that what really hit him was that people "weren't noticeably dying, or quickly dying, but dying cell by cell day by day, slow, lingering, with no hope."[10]

Glen Lake's philosophy of positive thinking presented sanatorium care as an opportunity for people to regain health. There were, in fact, a disproportionate number of tuberculosis survivors among doctors who worked in sanatoriums. At Glen Lake, that included doctors Frost, Jennings, Kinsella, Larson, Mattill, and Opstad. Tuberculosis survivors and others with health problems sought employment at sanatoriums because they offered a work schedule that incorporated regular rest hours and provided a healthful diet.

The doctors who had survived tuberculosis were among the most vocal advocates for following the rules and having a cheerful outlook. They believed that the proper attitude had served them well, and so they urged their own patients to do likewise.

Nurse Mary Shonka believed that attitude had something to do with survival. She told of a young person from Hopkins who was pessimistic about his life—so pessimistic that nothing would change his mind. "He was down, and he wasn't going to let you get him up," she said. And he died.

Manuel Martinez thought a fellow patient died because he was so afraid of surgery. He said, "I think that it wasn't the surgery that killed him. He was afraid of it and he died . . . Just didn't have the courage to go through with it."[11]

While some patients railed against the Pollyanna atmosphere pushed upon them, writings and interviews by many former Glen Lake patients point to a certain amount of success with that philosophy. Research on the role of the mind in health and healing that was once met with skepticism is now finding acceptance. Perhaps avoiding talk of death was not detrimental to long-term recovery, but instead was a form of cognitive-behavioral therapy ahead of its time.

Unless a roommate expired suddenly, patients rarely had personal experience of someone's demise. Most deaths occurred on the third floors. When someone died, their body would be unobtrusively moved to the sanatorium's morgue in East Basement. The morgue room featured a tall, two-door, refrigerated cooler encased in oak, resembling the ice boxes once found in homes. Even the kids in the Children's Building knew about the morgue. The older ones would scare the younger ones by telling them they were going past the morgue whenever they used the tunnels to travel to the main building, even though it was on a lower floor and none of them probably ever saw it.[12]

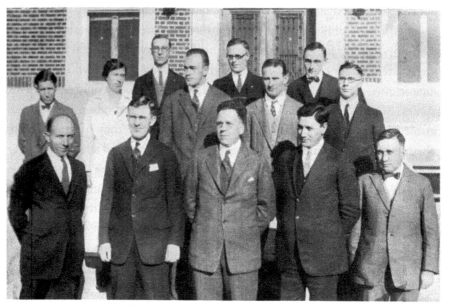

Physicians in 1920s. (Courtesy of the Lokke Collection)

Sanatoriums in Minnesota worked with local funeral homes, just as general hospitals did. Undertakers normally called for bodies at the ambulance entrance during rest hours from 1:30 to 2:30 p.m. and after 9:00 p.m. The entrance, at the back of the administration building, was not visible from patients' rooms. In the winter, undertakers were allowed to come between 6:00 and 7:00 p.m. "under cover of darkness." If it was necessary to come at other hours, the deceased would be transported to the power plant via the tunnel and would be picked up there.[13]

The sanatorium tried to cooperate as far as was possible and practical with special situations. The Minneapolis Jewish Orthodox Council informed the sanatorium that the Jewish religion did not permit the removal of a

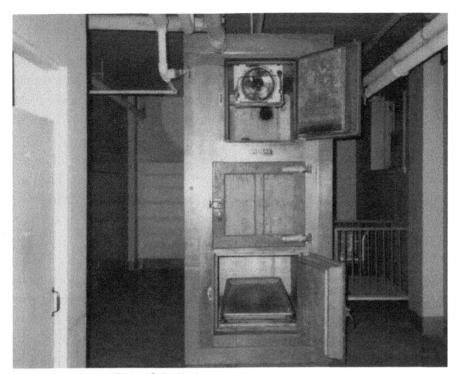

Morgue. (Courtesy of Barker Collection)

Jewish corpse on the Sabbath or on holiday except in extraordinary circumstances. The corpse of someone who died on a Saturday would be kept in the morgue until sundown of that day.[14]

The morgue was equipped for autopsies, and doctors sought to obtain postmortem examination permits from families. Families who gave permission for autopsies were helping to make future diagnoses more accurate. In the days before MRIs and ultrasounds, people who exhibited the symptoms of tuberculosis sometimes had complex medical issues, and an autopsy was often the only way to obtain that information. In addition, if a sanatorium wanted to be approved by the American Medical Association for residencies in tuberculosis, it needed to perform autopsies on at least fifteen percent of the patients who died.[15]

One autopsy in January 1933 revealed that a patient who seemed to have a textbook history of pulmonary tuberculosis really had a post-tonsillectomy pulmonary abscess.[16] In July of the same year, a person who returned to the sanatorium for the fourth time in eight years died. The autopsy confirmed tuberculosis, but he also had bronchiectasis, an obstructive lung disease for which a bronchoscopy to remove tissue might have been helpful.[17]

Other non-TB deaths included influenza, pneumonia, nephritis, and coronary sclerosis and thrombosis.[18] At the December 1933 medical meeting, a staff doctor reported a death from metastatic carcinoma of lungs. Even if it had been correctly diagnosed, there was no cure for cancer—successful chemotherapy was still years away.[19]

Also in 1933, a male patient who had been discharged earlier with healed tuberculosis of the hip was readmitted by his family practitioner. The sanatorium doctors found no tuberculosis, but treated the man by draining sinuses near his rectum. The autopsy found carcinoma of rectum, bladder, and prostate.[20]

Documentation of the information found during an autopsy had its challenges in the days before voice recorders and sophisticated photographic equipment. In the 1930s, Glen Lake employed artistic patient-employees in the Division of Illustration. The artists would produce plaster and wax models of tuberculous lesions in various organs of the body. Their work also included drawings of unusual lesions seen during operations and autopsies. These were later photographed and used on lantern slides to enable the physicians to present lectures to other staff. It was economical to have someone sketching because film was expensive. The estimated cost of illustration materials for 1933, including ink, Bristol board, paint, plaster, wax, pen, and crayons, was only fifteen dollars.[21] Helmer Gunnarson garnered special praise for his role as illustrator, although he preferred sculpting and could produce almost anything, including a full-sized skeleton.[22]

Even with humane care, the prospect of prolonged dying became too much for some patients to bear, and suicides did occur. The patient whose autopsy revealed multiple cancers took his own life. Without antibiotics and adequate pain relievers, his condition must have been unbearable. In 1927, a female patient jumped through a window on Three West, to the horror of roommates. Many patients, including Hannah Lokke, were awakened by the screams.[23]

In 1933, Jeff, one of the few black patients at Glen Lake also jumped from the third floor. A thirty-four-year-old widower who had been at Glen Lake for more than five years, he was buried at the Hennepin County Poor Farm.[24]

One of the deaths was unintentional. In 1938, a twenty-nine-year-old woman from Minneapolis attempted to leave the sanatorium via a third-floor window by climbing down a rope she had made from sheets tied together. The rope parted, and she fell to the ground. She died two days later.[25]

The saddest deaths by far were those of the youngest patients. Very few children actually died at the Children's Building, however. From the opening of the facility in 1922 until 1942, a total of fifteen children under the age of sixteen died. Of them, eleven perished from childhood-type, non-pulmonary tuberculosis. It seems to have been more common among the young patients than the adults, however, for them to be brought home

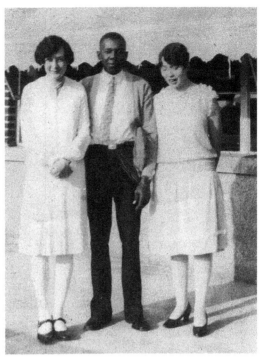

Patient, Jeff. (Courtesy of the Lokke Collection)

to die. Dr. Mariette noted in a 1937 report that a child discharged as unimproved was taken home by her parents because they were not permitted to visit her as often as they liked. The one child who died at Glen Lake that year was admitted with a tuberculous lesion on his hip. That condition might have responded to treatment, but he developed miliary tuberculosis and died after being in the Children's Building for 907 days.

Some children with active tuberculosis never resided with the other children. Dolores Romatko's younger brother, Jackie, had pulmonary tuberculosis and died in the main building when he was not quite two years old. His mother, Evelyn, was not allowed to attend Jackie's funeral because she was too ill at the time.[26]

At age one year and three months, Larry Botten came to Glen Lake from Montevideo, Minnesota. He had pulmonary tuberculosis and was admitted to the third floor in the main building. His father had survived tuberculosis, but three aunts died, including Ruby, who passed away at Glen Lake in the 1930s. Larry's grandparents had rented rooms to itinerant railroad workers,

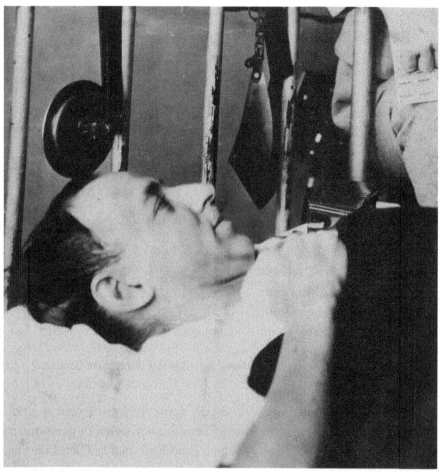

Patient with Sword of Damocles tied to his bed. (Courtesy of the Lokke Collection)

and it is believed that tuberculosis was introduced into the family by one or more of their boarders. Larry's family visited when they could, but he passed away in March 1945, 140 miles away from his home.[27]

One sanatorium couple was still grieving in the 1980s and reluctant to give their real names. "Alice" said she could see their young son, who was in the Children's Building, every ten days. "We were on litters. We'd look at each other through the (glass) door. He'd look at me and cry; I had to look at him and try not to cry. You did most of your crying at night." Her only son died. "Mentally, I think being in the san made it easier for us," she said. "A lot of people were dying. . . . I think that made it easier for us to accept."[28]

The underground nature of death topics created a well of dark humor at sanatoriums. Patients would have probably agreed with humorist Allen Klein, who said, "Humor can help you cope with the unbearable so that you can stay on the bright side of things until the bright side actually comes along." This was reflected in the content of the sanatorium newsletter. But subjects that were avoided in normal conversation showed up in other ways.

One example is the following ditty, meant to be sung to the tune of "My Bonnie Lies over the Ocean":

My father had tuberculosis, my mother had only one lung.
They spit up their blood in a bucket, and dried it and chewed it
for gum.
Dentyne, Dentyne, they dried it, and chewed it for gum, for gum.
Dentyne, Dentyne, they dried it, and chewed it for gum.

Because of a sanatorium's supposed dismal atmosphere of illness and death, several studies from the 1920s and 1930s stated that any optimism on the part of sanatorium patients was a compensation mechanism. They noted a form of disassociation or state of euphoria called "spes phthisica," which was present in advanced stages of the disease. Some authors claimed that "tuberculosis patients were self-centered, not interested in others, and somewhat reclusive." Others found that hypochondrias, anxiety, and depression were the prevailing moods.[29]

In 1941, a student at the University of Minnesota wanted to find out if those studies made valid observations. Did a sanatorium "personality" exist? Would patients respond differently from persons not in a sanatorium? As a student, Roger Page had access to an early version of the Minnesota Multiphasic Personality Inventory (MMPI). He administered it to several patients at Glen Lake as part of his thesis work for a doctorate degree.[30]

Based on the results of the MMPI, Page did see some deviations from the norm in areas of hypochondriasis, depression, and hysteria, with the first two being more elevated among males than females. He attributed this to the American culture and how tuberculosis limited men from performing their traditional roles of working and supporting others. He said his data did not support a "spes phthisica" and that, at Glen Lake at least, responses indicated attitudes of consideration and helpfulness, not self-centeredness.

Page concluded his report by suggesting that sanatorium staff could benefit from training in psychiatric and psychological specialties to help them better understand the patients and help them cope with illness and death.[31]

Dr. Mariette believed that if recovery was not possible, a sanatorium should be a place for people to receive good, humane care during their decline.[32] For that reason, chronically ill and incurable patients were granted exceptions to the rules, because strict adherence to the privilege system would mean never leaving their beds. Those who were able to be up and about were allowed a half hour of exercise out of doors, daily, although this did not allow them to go to the dining room. If they had attained full bathroom privileges and had been in the sanatorium at least five years total time, they were eligible for ten-hour leaves.[33] If a patient's prognosis was unfavorable, there was no limit put on the occupational craft work they did, except their own desire and ability to participate.[34]

In 1940, the medical staff recommended home care for Christopher T., a patient with an unfavorable prognosis. Dr. Mariette said that if an incoming patient was close to death, there was little to gain from admission to the sanatorium. "What is to be gained by separating them from their families just before death?" he asked, "Far better to engage a nurse and care for such cases in their homes rather than send them to a hospital or sanatorium to die."[35] Kübler-Ross addressed this in her book, too. Her plea for home care for the dying was an echo of Mariette's opinion forty years earlier.

As more patients survived and Glen Lake grew, so did the need for offering more than a bed for recovery and a book to read. The administrators knew it was difficult for people to leave behind an active, independent life and enter into the rigid routine of a sanatorium. When patients were very ill, they may have even derived comfort from the routine. Once they began to get well, however, they became bored and disruptive. Achieving a balance of rest and entertainment was a challenge discussed by doctors and administrators nationwide. Dr. Mariette had formed strong opinions about that balance, and he sought to create at Glen Lake an atmosphere that would produce what he called a "contented patient."

9

Contented Patients

B Y THE TIME THE CONSTRUCTION DUST settled at Glen Lake in 1924, Dr. Mariette oversaw the work and lives of more than 1,000 people. The bed count had increased to 417, but most of the state's 1,708 deaths from tuberculosis that year took place outside of a sanatorium. That was partly due to lack of capacity, but also to the reputation of sanatoriums as places to die.

In his book for patients, Dr. Pottenger attempted to dispel this reputation, writing,

> Some patients fear going to an institution because of a feeling that it is a gloomy and depressing place to be. The opposite is true. There is no happier or more cheerful set of optimists to be found anywhere than in a well-conducted sanatorium where patients are getting well of tuberculosis. It is a common experience that patients entering an institution are surprised at the general air of hopefulness and helpfulness and the lack of depressing influences.[1]

Dr. Mariette shared that point of view. Because the primary benefit of the institutions at that time was the removal of the infected person from society, it was important for him to create an atmosphere that welcomed and retained those with tuberculosis. Most people entered a sanatorium voluntarily and could leave without repercussion. In order to make them want to stay, Mariette considered every aspect of the sanatorium experience and made improvements.

In a report to the Hennepin County Sanatorium Commission, he said:

The great defect in our medical treatment of tuberculosis today lies in the fact that those responsible for the construction and maintenance of our institutions have not grasped the fact that from the standpoint of the medical and nursing care, and for the provision of a thorough clinical study of the cases, that the equipment and service of our sanatoria should resemble that of our best hospitals and not merely a first-class boarding home. The treatment to be effective should deal not with the lungs alone but with the entire patient.[2]

In 1926, he presented a paper to the Wisconsin Sanatorium Association at Muridale Sanatorium in Wawatosa. His speech, "Means of Promoting Contentment among Patients," summed up his philosophy that contentment was half the cure. Mariette began his presentation by comparing the sanatorium to a business. He noted that "good will" and public opinion were assets to the sanatorium, and the patients were the best "advertisers." It was everyone's responsibility to make the institution a place where patients wanted to go for treatment and where they would want to remain, he claimed. He described how Glen Lake Sanatorium provided several services that contributed to contentment.[3]

All new patients were admitted through the social service department. Social worker Lanore Ward had been succeeded in 1921 by Marguerite Ridler, and the duties no longer included entertaining the patients. Customer service began when someone from the department contacted the patient at home, before admission to the sanatorium, and a complete social history was obtained.

Part of the admission process was a frank talk with the patient to explain the rigid rules, because the way they were presented affected the degree to which they were followed. Patients were told about the two "Rs" of sanatorium life: rest and regulation. It was imperative for new patients to understand that the cost of getting well was strict adherence to a resting routine believed to be beneficial for people with tuberculosis. A favorite saying of the admissions staff was, "heaven and the sanatorium help those who help themselves, but neither heaven nor the sanatorium can help an unwilling patient."[4]

The patients' needs were considered, and a program was developed that suported both the mental and physical aspects of hospitalization. The social

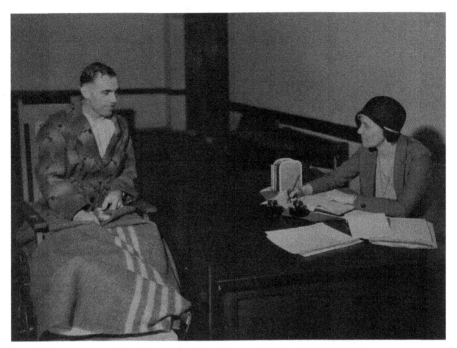

Social Services consulting. (Courtesy of the Minnesota Historical Society)

worker consulted with the education department to create an educational plan if needed.

The social services department contacted the patient's family and attempted to help them with their worries about food, rent, or clothing. Carl Wilwerding's stay at Glen Lake was typical of the upheaval caused when the wage earner was absent in an era when most middle-class women did not work. During Carl's confinement, his wife, Wilhelmina, began working as a furrier for Ribnik Furs in Minneapolis to support the family. Their son and one daughter were sent to California to live with their uncle for a year, while an older daughter remained in Minnesota.[5]

Once family issues had been addressed by social services, and the patient was settled into a bed, other factors in the sanatorium's campaign for contentment came into play.

Food service was uppermost in the plan for improved health. Dr. Mariette summarized the sanatorium's efforts in a paper titled "The Food Problem in a Sanatorium" and acknowledged that food and diet played an important role in the treatment of a disease so frequently associated with weight loss.[6]

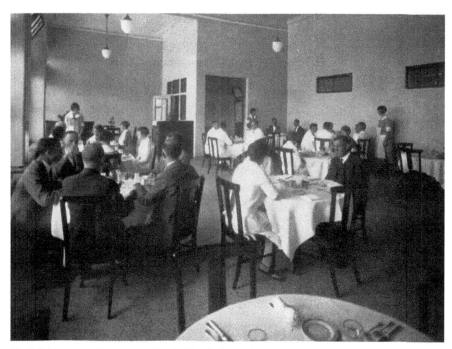

Staff dining room. (Courtesy of the Lokke Collection)

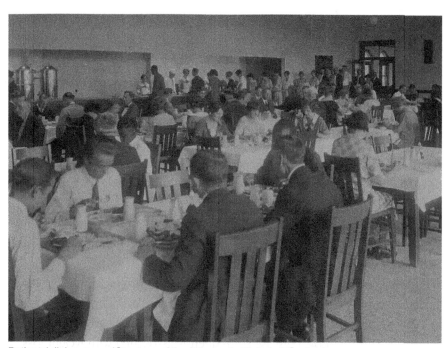

Patients' dining room. (Courtesy of the Minnesota Historical Society)

Dr. J.A. Myers, professor of medicine at the University of Minnesota, agreed. "Nothing results in more dissatisfaction among patients than insufficient, poorly prepared or improperly served food. . . . Patients themselves have known best the great importance of cooks in sanatoriums. It is the cooks who have made the food palatable and thus have kept many patients in sanatoriums who otherwise would have left against advice."[7]

Serving a large variety of food properly cooked and seasoned is always a challenge in a large institution. Functioning primarily as a long-term hospital, the sanatorium also needed to prepare special diets for persons with complications such as diabetes, gastric and duodenal ulcers, tuberculosis of the intestinal tract, and hypertension. The patients were also varied in their religions, allergies, culture preferences, and eating habits.

In the 1920s, nutrition as a profession was in its infancy. The American Dietetic Association had just been formed in 1917, and it wasn't until the passage of the federal Maternity and Infancy Protection Act in 1921 that state health boards were allowed to hire nutritionists. Sanatoriums like Glen Lake, with their large and relatively stable populations, invested considerable effort into learning how to develop nutritious yet economical meals to improve the health of their patients.

By 1928, the Glen Lake kitchen staff was serving between 600 and 700 patients at each meal, plus employees. In those days, a strong organizational hierarchy dictated the eating arrangements. The doctors' dining room was "holy territory" used only by the upper administrators, and they were waited on by maids. The remaining six dining rooms were for patients, staff nurses, student nurses, dietary employees, male employees, and female employees.[8]

Non-ambulant East- and West-Wing and Main-Building patients ate in bed or at their bedside. The formal third-floor dining room—with its large windows, skylight, tablecloths, and cloth napkins—provided a welcoming atmosphere for the patients. It was one of the few places where men and women could mingle, and it played an important part in the system of privileges. When a newly semi-ambulant person came in, the other diners rattled their dishes to celebrate.[9]

Lucille Townsend, director of household, decided that the kitchen would not serve the same menu throughout the institution. The nine-day dinner (noon meal) schedule that she implemented was divided among nine units of service with five rotating menus for patients and four for employees.

This made it possible to serve foods that could not be easily prepared for 600 or 700 people at the same time. Entrées could be roast beef, steak, liver or bacon, roast lamb, lamb stew, ham, veal roast, pork chops, or chicken.[10]

This rotating plan also meant that no one received the same meat on the same day on two successive weeks. The serving of side dishes was planned in the same manner so each entrée was paired with either scalloped, mashed, or boiled potatoes. Vegetables, relishes, desserts, and bakery goods were added last, and factors such as color, flavor, and dryness were considered when planning the menu.

In addition, Townsend initiated a modified selective menu, something that didn't become common in many hospitals until the 1980s. The staff dieticians interviewed new patients about their preferences, especially with fish and lamb. The kitchen served a lutefisk dinner at Christmas, and dietitians had to find out who wanted lutefisk and who didn't. Cheese and eggs were always available as an option for patients who didn't like certain foods. The established rotating menu made it possible for patients to plan ahead and request substitutions in advance. One nurse on each floor was designated as the diet nurse to handle requests and complaints. Dr. Mariette acknowledged the initial labor involved in creating the plan, but he pointed out that preparation, waste, and after-work had been reduced.

The kitchen's food carts were electrically heated and carried hot foods directly from the kitchen to the floors. Trays were pre-readied with bread and cold foods in the serving rooms on each floor. Working for the dietary department was Juanita Fleury Seck's first job as a nineteen-year-old, and her duty was to make sure patients got the correct special diet trays. She also had to set each tray with knife, fork, spoon, and a cloth napkin.[11]

Because the hot food was dished up at the bedsides, patients could choose the portion size of their meals. "Nothing does more to gain the confidence and support of the patient than the feeling that he is an individual and that in so far as possible his opinion will be considered," said Mariette about food service.

Frederick Manfred believed that his stomach would help him win his battle against TB.

> My stomach would win out for me because I could eat anytime, anywhere, and almost everything. . . . Johnny the orderly would

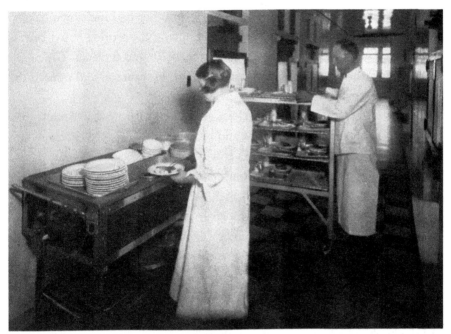

Food services. (Courtesy of the Lokke Collection)

come by in the morning, and after he finished the whole floor, he knew I always liked seconds. He opened the door and he said, "Seconds today?" And I said, "Yeah, what have you got out there?" One morning, "Oh," he says, "I've got seventeen eggs." I said, "Bring them in here." I ate them all.[12]

The food given to patients had a high protein value and calorie count to build new tissue and keep patients from losing weight. Wilton Lofstrand, a patient, kept track of the food delivered on his tray for one week, plus he took second helpings for four breakfasts. His average calorie count by meal was: breakfast—834, dinner—753, and supper—779, for a daily average of 2,349 calories. If he had eaten only what came on his tray, the average would have been 2,200 calories, which is approximately what the dietitians planned for.[13]

The employees were well fed, too. They were exposed to active tuberculosis during work, and if they weren't healthy they could be more susceptible to developing it themselves. "Skinny" was a bad word. Lage Floren, a patient for two and a half years and later an employee in the print shop, said, "The food was very good. They had good cooks, and they had their own bakery. Some people said they had the best doughnuts in the world."[14] Lyl Borak, who started working at the sanitorium in the 1920s and replaced Townsend as household director in the 1940s, agreed with his opinion and praised the baker, James Egan.[15]

"We ate well," remembered Deloise Anderson Clair who, like many other staff members, lived on campus and received meals as part of room and board. Those who lived off-campus could pay to eat there, too. Clair particularly remembers the delicious shrimp jambalaya—rice with jumbo shrimp on top.[16]

The sanatorium had its own garden for a while, but it became impractical to plan menus around the abundance of vegetables that ripened at the same time. Gardening ceased and in-season vegetables were purchased at a farmer's market once a week.[17] Canned goods were selected through an anonymous bid process that included taste-testing of contents with labels removed from the cans. Beef was stored for three weeks so it would be aged, and the kitchen had its own butcher shop.[18]

Glen Lake also had its own garbage disposal system starting in 1922: a piggery. Food scraps from the kitchen were collected and taken over to a

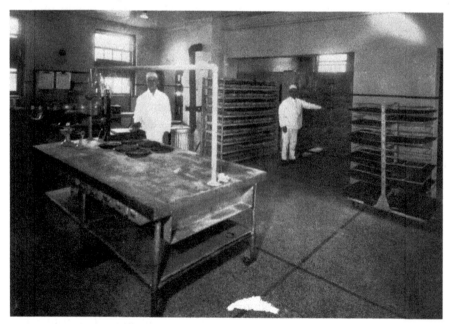

The bakery. (Courtesy of the Lokke Collection)

building behind the power house. The garbage was cooked in a kettle and served to the pigs, which were later sold. Charles Sampson, who managed the facility operations, said that making 100-pound pigs into 250-pound hogs at the rate of 120 per year with no cost for food brought in money.[19]

The dietary department obtained milk from a herd at the nearby Glen Lake Farm School for Boys. The kitchen staff then pasteurized and bottled the milk and churned butter. This action was prompted by the threat of herd-to-human transmission of bovine tuberculosis. In 1904, tests at the Phipps Institute in Pennsylvania confirmed that tuberculosis could be transmitted from cows to people.[20] Studies by other researchers showed that "tubercle bacilli may be contained in all the products of milk, cheese, butter, whey, and skim milk."[21] Walter Parks Raymond, a former butter maker, had died at Glen Lake on May 28, 1916, after being there about one month. Raymond suffered with tuberculosis for fifteen years. It is possible that his occupational exposure to milk products resulted in his disease.[22]

Minnesota's Live Stock Sanitary Board was among the first nationally to regulate the shipment and testing of livestock based on a suspected link. Unfortunately, the cost of testing a herd and reimbursing farmers for destroyed animals was large. Milk producers and politicians had an economic incentive to question the link between cows and people, and they sought to halt testing.[23]

Additional studies reported on the efficacy of destroying tuberculosis bacilli by heating milk. Minnesota's State Medical Association recommended the sterilization of milk at 160 degrees as a way to arrest the progress of the disease. This met opposition from farmers who protested the extra expense, from doctors who questioned the destruction of all germs, and from consumers who said they didn't like the taste of the milk. Most health boards acted cautiously, and it would be decades before the practice of testing herds, pasteurizing milk, and destroying tuberculous cows became routine. Glen Lake ensured the quality of its dairy products by doing its own processing.[24]

Food was important for contentment. So was mental stimulation, and by 1925, there were approximately 3,000 books in the library. Edith Corson was assigned to work in the library that year and eventually became employed as the head librarian. Corson said, "The immediate aim was the therapeutic one of contentment and guided mental occupation, and the long-range one was to make lifelong readers, since it is the ideal recreation for the tuberculous."

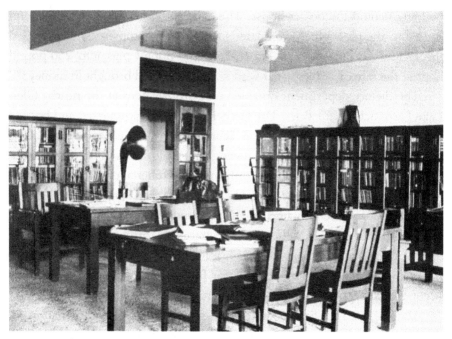

The library. (Courtesy of the Lokke Collection)

Another idea for creating a satisfied state of mind involved occupational therapy to keep idle hands busy. For most sanatoriums, occupational therapy meant light hobby crafts such as needlework done to pass the time. Nopeming Sanatorium was first to introduce occupational therapy for tuberculous patients in Minnesota, and Glen Lake was the second, with those duties combined with social services until Gracia Loehl was employed as director of a separate department.

Dr. Mariette believed patients should sell what they made, if they wished, and receive the profit. Earning even a small bit of income would give them money to spend at the sanatorium store or to send home to help with expenses.[25] This controversial idea was debated at conferences and in medical journals. Doctors feared that some sanatoriums used occupational therapy to get work done more cheaply at the sanatorium. The greatest notoriety was attached to the municipal sanatorium at Otisville, New York, which put patients to work as part of their course of treatment, often just weeks after admission.[26] Other doctors believed that the thought of financial gain could encourage patients to take on too much work, which could then hamper their recovery.

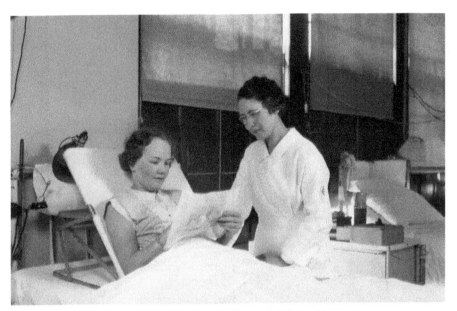

Occupational therapy woman. (Courtesy of the Hennepin History Museum)

The system at Glen Lake ensured that occupational therapy was primarily craft work approved by a physician, but that products could be sold if the patient wanted to earn a small income. Occupational therapy clearly differed from light physical labor, which consisted of unpaid chores assigned as part of the work-up leading to discharge.

The tradition of displaying occupational therapy products at the Hennepin County and Minnesota State fairs continued for decades, as did the sale of articles at the sanatorium, local bazaars, and Dayton's and Donaldson's department stores in Minneapolis.[27]

One patient made a lot of potholders because they sold easily. She also made soakers (covers for cloth diapers).[28] Another made yarn pictures and also crafted sequin earrings to make some money. She charged a dollar a pair for those earrings and could make four pairs a day. A friend of hers made shell earrings to sell.[29]

Men did handicrafts, too. Kenneth Berg learned leather craft at the sanatorium. In later years, he employed this skill to do custom tooling on show saddles.[30] George and Jack, two men on Four East, worked on luncheon cloths using an intricate and traditional Norwegian style of embroidery known as hardanger.[31]

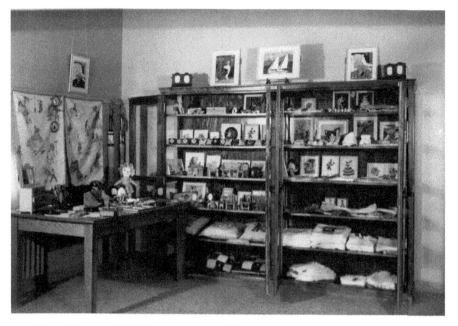

Patients' craftwork for sale. (Courtesy of the Hennepin History Museum)

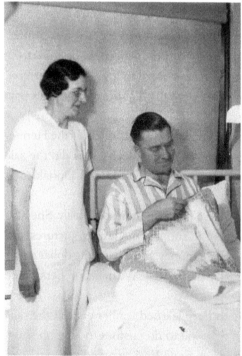

More occupational therapy. (Courtesy of the Hennepin History Museum)

Manuel Martinez remembered his work on the Lord's Prayer in the Garden of Eden. "10,000 cross stitches," he said. "When it was finished, the frame cost about $2.50, which at that time was expensive. . . . They offered me fifty bucks. I figured out that with all the time I put into it, it would come out to about four cents an hour. I've got it yet," he said when interviewed.[32]

By the 1920s, everything offered for sale was sterilized to remove the danger of transmitting tubercle bacilli. Sterilization of occupational therapy items included washing, ironing, or using an autoclave (high-pressure saturated steam). The making of anything that would hold articles intended to be put in the mouth, such as leather cigarette cases, was discontinued. Other types of leather work and wood carving were distributed without sterilization or put under the alpine lamp for one hour.[33]

Dr. Mariette, whose family attended church, believed that spiritual comfort was also important to the plan for contentment. On Sundays, the auditorium served as a sanctuary for regular church services. The Elks Lodge No. 44 of Minneapolis donated an oak altar that was moved in front of the stage each week.[34]

Pastor Edwin Kurth from Zion Lutheran in Hopkins initiated weekly services. He was later succeeded by pastors Carl Mundinger, Walter Clausen, and Eugene Seltz. Catholic parishes conducted Mass each Sunday, and chaplains included Father Francis Fleming, Father Francis Hays, and Father Thomas Jude.[35] Father Fleming remembered the warm welcome he received, no matter what the patient's denomination, and the caring nurses who needed to call him in the middle of the night to administer sacraments to the dying. All pastors were required to take a TB skin test occasionally, wear a white gown when visiting the floors, and observe sanitary procedures, such as hand washing. Fleming also remembered the anxiety he felt when he had an extended cold and the relief after a chest X-ray turned out to be negative for tuberculosis.[36]

Several area churches maintained a relationship with Glen Lake throughout the years of operation and conducted services. They included St. Joseph's Catholic in Hopkins, Immaculate Heart of Mary in Minnetonka, and Calvary Baptist and Grace Presbyterian in Minneapolis. Reverend Elliot Marston from St. Stephen's Episcopal Church in Edina was a frequent visitor to his parishioners.

Several former patients mentioned the role of faith in their process of healing. Oscar Eliason and his brother Paul became patients in 1929, soon after Oscar's graduation from the Northwestern Bible and Missionary Training School. After Paul's death, Oscar was discouraged and requested an evangelical minister to come to Glen Lake and pray for him with a laying-on of hands. When Oscar was discharged, he began a life of music evangelism and composition. His song, "Got Any Rivers," became a camp revival favorite and was recorded by gospel singer Mahalia Jackson.[37]

There was apparently no specific service to the Jewish patients until Rabbi Milton Kopstein was hired as a state chaplain to serve Minnesota's state institutions in about 1950. Jewish patients relied on several service organizations for visits. For a short while an organization of young Jewish women, known as Junior Aid, raised money to buy clothing and gifts for Jewish residents. The differing Sabbath days, Saturday and Sunday, as well as the issue of kosher food, made it challenging for the sanatorium to make accommodations. The kitchen attempted to meet dietary restrictions and often failed. This issue, plus requests for leaves to observe Jewish holidays,

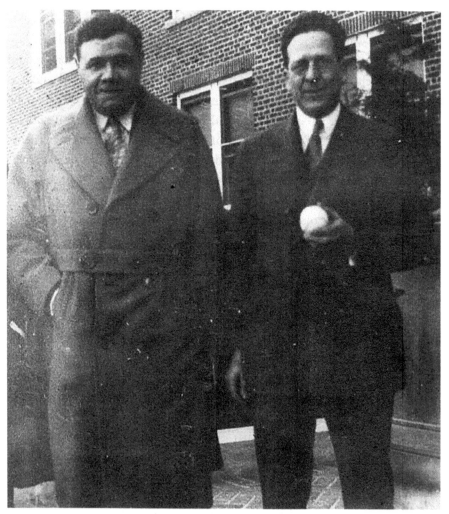

Babe Ruth visits Glen Lake Sanatorium. (Courtesy of the Lokke Collection)

was occasionally a topic of discussion at medical staff meetings. When asked for an opinion on someone's requests for Passover, Dr. Cohen replied that when people are sick the Jewish rules for holidays don't apply.[38]

Celebrities were brought to the sanatorium in an attempt to lift spirits. The most famous may have been Yankee baseball player George Herman (Babe) Ruth. He took a break from a performance in Minneapolis and visited the sanatorium in 1926, the year he hit a record three runs in the World Series.[39] Charles Lindberg, "Lucky Lindy," circled the sanatorium in the *Spirit of St. Louis* on August 24, 1927, before heading to the Lindbergh home in Little Falls.[40]

The Shriners established a relationship with Glen Lake and played an important part in the social activities. Groups would come out accompanied by a male chorus or a clown, who walked throughout the building to entertain folks. They also booked entertainers to perform in the auditorium.[41]

There always seemed to be something going on at Glen Lake. In smaller institutions, far from major population centers and with fewer social distractions, an extended stay at a sanatorium was often boring and monotonous. Dr. Mariette was able to institute several of his plans because Glen Lake was near to a major metropolitan area. The economic and community resources for the much-needed distractions were nearby. This was especially apparent in the many forms of entertainment the patients enjoyed.

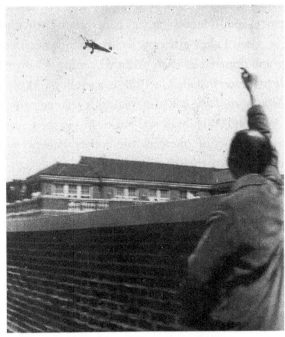

Charles Lindbergh visit. (Courtesy of the Lokke Collection)

10

Entertainment

D IVERSIONS AND ENTERTAINMENTS of all types formed an important aspect of Dr. Mariette's plan for patients. He summed up this particular philosophy in a 1927 article published in *The Modern Hospital*: "We attempt to give them as good a time as they can stand."[1]

Dr. J.P. Murphy, who was a patient at Glen Lake, recognized the need for distractions. He said that the constant emphasis upon the state of the body could result in a preoccupation very close to hypochondria. The microscopic living situation could cause trivialities to assume disproportionate importance, and, therefore, it was necessary to provide diversions.[2]

Glen Lake's attempts to keep minds occupied started with that phonograph donated in 1916. Another significant distraction arrived when a radio system was installed in 1921 as a result of $1,800 donated by readers of the *Minneapolis Journal*. Radio was still a relatively new medium at that time. Only about 600,000 homes and businesses in the United States had radios, and the average cost of one was fifty dollars. Patients now had access to a medium that many of their families lacked.[3]

The system at Glen Lake collected radio impulses via an aerial. Those radio impulses were changed by three radio sets into electrical impulses. Wires led from each radio set to corresponding outlets by each bed in the building. It was basically a telephone system with the radio set talking into one end and the listener hearing the conversation or music at the other. One outlet was for in-house broadcasts and the other two were for local AM radio stations KSTP and WCCO. The system was an important contact with the outside world because the patients were not supposed to bring in their own radios or to use any amplifiers.[4,5]

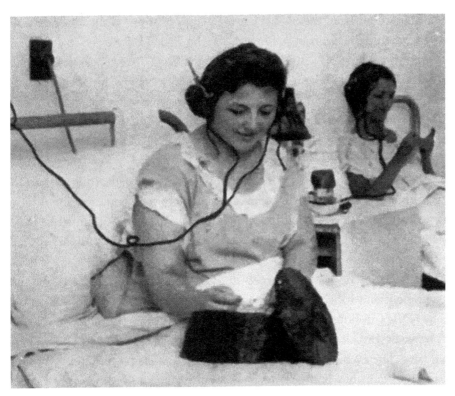

Patient with radio system. (Courtesy of the Lokke Collection)

Alfred Greene, a University of Minnesota student who had been pursuing an engineering degree before being admitted to Glen Lake, wondered about the possibilities of hijacking the radio system with his contraband amplifier. He rigged up a microphone transmitter and plugged it into the socket used for in-house broadcasts. He said, "Hello," and the next day he received a note telling him that his voice was heard very clearly. Al went on the air every night after nine o'clock to tell jokes and stories.

His clandestine radio show came to the attention of administration, and

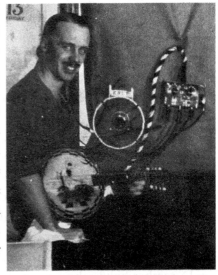

Al Greene on KNUT radio. (Courtesy of the Lokke Collection)

Dr. Mariette ordered the broadcasting to stop. Al went on the air one more night and told the listeners to request that the station be allowed to continue. Within three days, Mariette's office received about 350 letters asking for the show to go on. He relented and allowed a short evening broadcast during rest hour. Because stations west of the Mississippi River begin their call letters with a K and because Oak Terrace had a connection to acorns and because the whole operation seemed a bit nutty, KNUT was adopted for the identification letters.[6]

KNUT station was the first in-house hospital broadcasting system in the United States, and other hospitals and sanatoriums inquired about how it was set up. Waverly Sanatorium in Louisville, Kentucky, claimed to have had the first radio system, but theirs was a single signal only. It didn't supply three radio stations to patients until 1957.[7,8]

When Greene was discharged in 1928, the Trudeau Club bought the equipment and took on radio broadcasting as one of the club's functions. The KNUT in-house connection was used for morning announcements and for weekly broadcasts by the medical staff about tuberculosis and related updates. The evening announcers were male patients up on exercise. During each program they had time to play about eighteen 78-rpm records along with making calendar announcements. They received an average of thirty requests for each program.[9]

Although KNUT was an important source of amusement and information, its air time was limited to a few hours each day. The library, on the other hand, provided a more accessible activity. Patients on full-exercise privileges brought a library cart to patient floors. Readers could choose among the many newspapers delivered throughout the building: *The Minneapolis Morning Tribune*, the *Minneapolis Daily Times*, the *Minneapolis Star Journal*, and the *Minneapolis Sunday Tribune and Star Journal*. There were also books and more than seventy magazines they could choose to read. Most patients gave up reading books about TB, though, because as patient Elsie Hestevold said, "Every book says that the victim remains cheerful and hopeful to the very end."[10]

The Christmas holidays provided another diversion that was the highlight of the year. A lucky few patients got leaves to go home for the holidays, but in reality there were some patients who would never go home. For them, the December holiday became an extravaganza that contained all of their future Christmases.

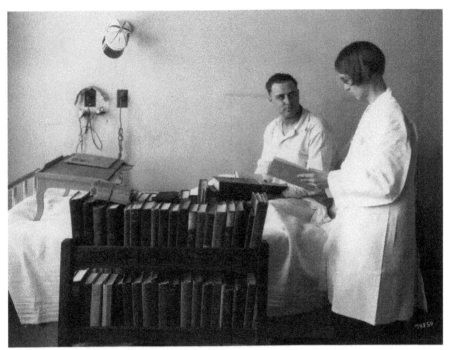

Library cart. (Courtesy of the Hennepin Museum)

In its first years of operation, the sanatorium's cottage population was small enough for patients to have a family-style celebration. On Christmas Eve they gathered around a decorated tree in the dining room. Under the tree went the gifts mailed to them from friends and relatives. Names were exchanged and each patient also wrapped an inexpensive gift for another patient, so no one went without a present to unwrap. As the sanatorium expanded, an attempt was made to continue with the distribution of gifts on Christmas Eve, but the sheer volume of packages made it impossible.[11]

The Shriners could always be counted on to bring excitement for the holidays, and Christmas 1934 was "the outstanding event of the year" thanks to their presence.

The Shriners hosted two parties. One was in the afternoon for the children, with Santa and a present for each child along with apples, oranges, candy, and nuts. The evening party for adults included the Shrine Funmakers (clowns) roaming through the sanatorium.

The highlight was entertainment in the auditorium by
• the Zurah Temple Band under the direction of Mr. Rossiter,
• the Zurah Temple Chanters under the direction of William MacPhail,

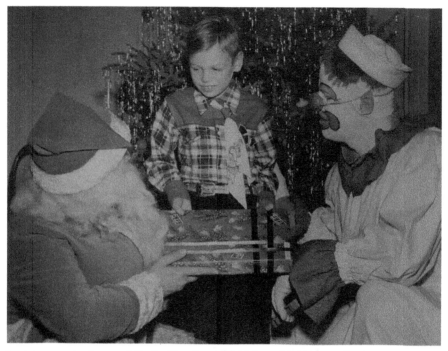

Christmas party clown and Santa. (Courtesy of the Minnesota Historical Society)

- the Woodward Sisters presenting saxophone and banjo numbers,
- Art Johnson, magician, with rabbits,
- Grace Spencer with ballet numbers,
- Lang and Lee, comedy jugglers,
- Grace Hubner, a prominent Northwest harpist, and
- Chief Chibiabos, a Chippewa singing to harp accompaniment.

The youngsters at the Children's Building had all the hoopla at Christmas that the adults did, and more. LuDean Harmsen Pontius remembers:

In the wards, we hung our stockings at the end of the beds, right on the foot of the bed. I'm sure there were a lot of toys donated, because I never had any family that sent me toys. I'd get one or two from my mother and from my dad when he was alive earlier. At night we'd all go to sleep all excited with one eye open and in the morning the stocking would be all full of stuff. At the very bottom of the sock there would always be a special toy and then

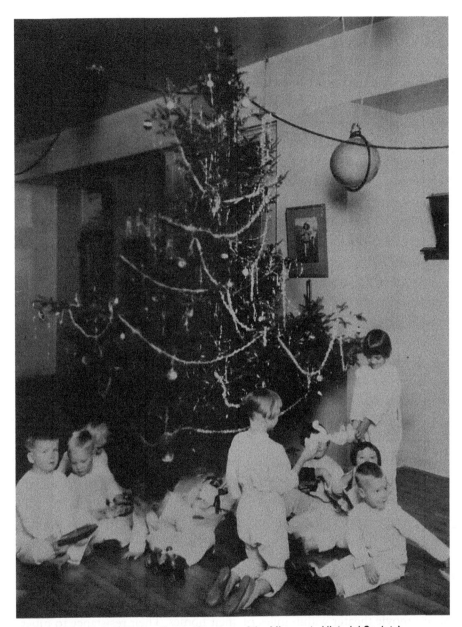

Christmas tree and children patients. (Courtesy of the Minnesota Historical Society)

the rest was filled with nuts and apples and oranges right up to the top. Then under the bed you'd have your big box. You'd get out, and you'd pull your box out and in there were all these wrapped presents. I'll bet you each child got ten wrapped presents.[12]

The youngsters in the Children's Building had three Christmas parties that year. In addition to the Shriners, they were entertained by visitors from St. Therese Catholic Church in Minnetonka and the Swedish Tabernacle, which was on the corner of Seventh and Chicago in Minneapolis.[13]

Other holidays were not slighted, either. Some years, the Catholic Women's Hospital Association or Zion Lutheran Church Women hosted Easter parties for female patients and gave them packages of cookies.[14] On Easter Day, patients held an Easter parade of sorts, with new bedclothes making an appearance at breakfast or during morning church services.

Halloween was livened up with decorations throughout the building and the telling of horror stories featuring the tunnels and the morgue. One year the elevator by the dining room was turned into a chamber of horrors. Beef bones from the kitchen hung from the ceiling.[15]

Another tradition that continued from the first cottages into the new building was movie night. The auditorium contained several rows of wooden movie-theater seats, but the majority of the large hall remained empty to make room for wheelchairs and litters. Someone from the sanatorium drove into Minneapolis each Wednesday morning to pick up films. Members of Minneapolis's Movie Projector's Union came out on a volunteer basis to run the equipment. A separate projection room at the back of the auditorium could be reached by a narrow inside staircase or an exterior door. The audience saw only silent films for many years because the sanatorium didn't have money in the budget to upgrade the projectors for talking films.[16]

Dora Cohen remembered the weekly movies as a gala social event, writing, "I will never forget the sight of that auditorium filled to capacity with litters, wheelchairs, and ambulatory patients."[17] Children from the summer camp across the road could also attend the Wednesday night shows because they already tested positive for tuberculosis. They sat in a group separate from the adults. Neighborhood children liked movie night, too, and tried to sneak into the sanatorium. It was a big temptation for children who didn't have a movie theater within miles of their homes. Their resistance to tuberculosis was unknown, so guards stood at the doors to keep them out for their own safety. Otherwise, they could be contaminated when they hid in areas considered unclean.[18]

Vaudeville acts traveling the United States often came out to provide entertainment. The Hans Kasemann Midgets made an appearance in 1927.

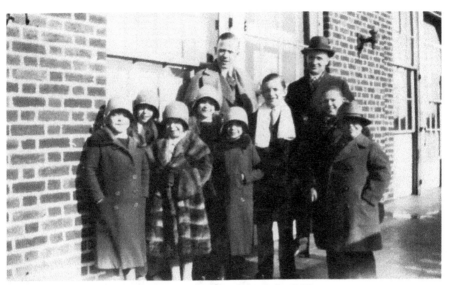

The Hans Kasemann Midgets. (Courtesy of the Lokke Collection)

Some vaudevillians came to stay. Fawn Lynn, a dancer from Minneapolis named Florence Morse at birth, traveled the national circuit. Her roving career included an appearance at the Empress in St. Paul with her husband, Emmett, in 1924. She spent three years at Glen Lake, while her husband pursued a career in Hollywood. *Terrace Topics* referred to her as the patient with the most beautiful name. Lynn regarded her stay at Glen Lake as an "indefinite run."[19]

Another pastime was the bane of any community: gossip. Medical staff regarded it as a source of misinformation and fear mongering. Patients who carried papers, passed milk, and did other odd jobs about the floors were told to stop spreading depressing gossip about other patients.[20] The telling of stories about people who had died was hard to control, whether they were true or false.

In keeping with customs at other institutions, such as colleges and boarding schools, new arrivals were sometimes subjected to hazing rituals. One patient had a hemorrhage shortly after being frightened during an episode of hazing.[21]

Patients also played tricks to pass the time, and student nurses were a favorite target. One of Phyllis Burns's assignments as a student nurse was to bring patients to the operating room. Instead of checking with the charge nurse, she went to the ward and asked for the patient by name. One of the

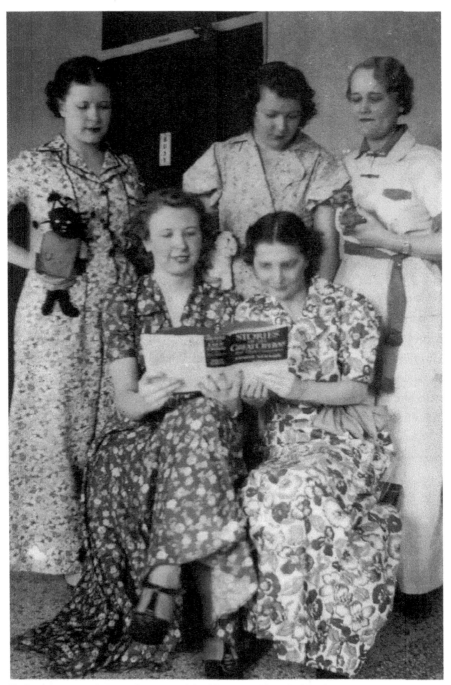

Patients in pretty clothes. (Courtesy of the Minnesota Historical Society)

men said, "That's me." She wheeled him to the operating room, but it was the wrong patient. The operating room nurse sent her back, and again she returned with the wrong person. The nurse disciplined her for showing poor judgment, and the men who had teased her felt so bad about their deception they had a dozen roses delivered to her.[22]

Don Martin remembered the initiations to which his ward mates subjected student nurses. Whenever new students came they asked them to go to the supervisor and get a pneumogauge stretcher. This was a practical joke, a wild goose chase, like looking for a left-handed monkey wrench.[23]

Some female patients spent a lot of time on their appearance. Nurse Mary Shonka said women became more beautiful after they were in the sanitorium for a while. They had time to think about fashions and work on their hair and manicures.[24] Lucille Saan's stepmother claimed that when she came to Glen Lake to visit, she felt like she was in Hollywood. The women dressed up in fancy negligees, and everyone looked so wonderful.[25] Newcomers said that it was easy to tell the visitors from the patients, because the visitors all looked sick.[26]

Creative rule-breaking was another pastime. Patients tamed squirrels by offering them food through the windows, which was against the rules. Occasionally a squirrel wanted more than was offered and tore through a screen and wreaked havoc in a room.[27]

Ambulant patients especially had opportunities for mischief. One patient had a pass for the weekend, but he was not supposed to be out at any public place. Unwisely, he went to a football game. Unfortunately, his seat was right next to Dr. Fenger.[28]

A male patient on Four Administration had a twin brother. One time on visiting day, the twins exchanged clothes and the patient went out for an unofficial leave. The nurses didn't hear about that until much later.[29]

Some patients made use of their free time for correspondence. They wrote letters and sent cards to friends and family members. Some acquired pen pals in other sanatoriums, even in other countries. There was also thriving intra-sanatorium note-writing. Patients who were on strict bed kept in touch with fellow patients via mail. Postal regulations required that envelopes handled by the post office needed a stamp, even with the addressee in the same building, so patients, not wanting to suffer that expense, relied on obliging nurses and orderlies to deliver their mail. Parents in the main building wrote letters to offspring in the Children's Building, which cost one cent to mail because the post office personnel couldn't handle unstamped mail. Eventually, arrangements were made for a stamp-free direct delivery.[30]

Visitors were both a welcome distraction and a boost to the spirit. Mariette's administrative philosophy encouraged and maintained relatively generous visiting hours compared with many sanatoriums that limited visits to Sundays only. In 1925, the medical staff decided to establish visiting times for every afternoon from 3:15 to 5:00 p.m. and also in the evening after rest hour was over at 7:00 p.m. There were still limits, however. Patients could either have three or four visitors for ten minutes each or one visitor for half an hour.[31]

Even the most welcome of visitors could unintentionally irritate the patients. A common pet peeve was the inevitable comment about rest: "Oh boy, I'd sure like to be able to lie around all day and not do anything but read movie magazines." Patients laughed it off but after a while it got old.[32] Don Rivers, a patient, wrote tongue-in-cheek rules for visiting:

- Always greet patient with "You don't look sick, what are you doing in bed?"
- Follow with "Move over and let me lie down beside you." Or, "Lucky devil! What I wouldn't give to trade places with you."
- Never sit closer than ten feet.
- Be sure to tell the patient in glamorous detail about the simply wonderful time you've been having. End with "We've all thought of you so often and wished you could have joined the fun."
- Try a little uplift work. "What are you complaining about? You have a roof over your head and three square meals a day. What more do you want?"
- When meal trays arrive, "My, that looks good! Makes me hungry to watch you. Can't you get another fork and let me join in?"
- Never leave the patient without calling his attention at least once to the lovely view outside his window. Conclude with, "I'll bet you never tire of it."
- Drop in on a patient and look startled and ask, "What? You still here?"

• Be generous in buying delicacies for patient—especially where highly perishable foods are concerned.

• Write a card or letter saying you'll be out to see him definitely on such-and-such an afternoon or evening. Forget about engagement completely; don't show up.[33]

Organizations and social groups were encouraged to tour the sanatorium and see firsthand what the institution was doing in the fight against tuberculosis. In November 1922, thirty-eight members of the Women's Club of Lake Minnetonka visited and were impressed with what they saw. They were shown the kitchen and laundry, led through the tunnels, and treated to tea in the nurses' dining room after walking through parts of the main building. In an article written for the *Excelsior–Minnetonka Record*, one of the club members said, "Many shrink from the idea of visiting the patients but this feeling passes once you have seen how cheerful and happy they are." Although it's quite probable that patients were prepped for the tourists, Dr. Mariette's primary intent was to demystify the institution and make the growing neighborhood feel comfortable with having a colony of tuberculous people in its midst.[34]

In 1925, the sanatorium hosted editors from Hennepin County's newspapers to give them a close-up view of the buildings and the methods of caring for and treating patients. The editor of the *Hopkins Review* later informed his readers that they would benefit from a visit to the place. He praised the people of Hennepin County for expending the funds necessary to build the sanatorium and equip it with thoroughly modern equipment. He also noted Dr. Mariette's wish to "make the Glen Lake institution the best in the country."

Later that month, it was the Girls and Boys Club of School District No. 38 who were treated to a presentation by the medical staff. The sanatorium staff also took part in publicity campaigns for local Christmas seal sales. Unfortunately, Dr. Mariette had to warn the public that a fake solicitor was selling seals and pictures and claiming that the funds were for Glen Lake, when no one was authorized to do so.[35]

Traveling to the sanatorium for a visit was no simple jaunt. In the early years, individual car ownership was still a rarity. In the 1920s, most visitors traveled from Minneapolis on the Minnetonka streetcar line. The most common route was from Hopkins on Excelsior Boulevard to the Glen Lake streetcar intersection and then south on a gravel road (known as Eden Prairie Road). In 1921, it cost staff and visitors twenty-four cents to ride the streetcar, and then they were responsible for making arrangements for the wagon or sleigh to get to the sanatorium from Glen Lake Station. A shuttle bus added in 1924 improved the journey to the sanatorium.[36]

Deloise Anderson Clair may have been influenced in her later career as a nurse at Glen Lake by her visits to her older brother, who was a patient there from 1929 to 1932. She and her mother traveled out on the streetcar from Minneapolis, but she recalled that the trip all the way out to Glen Lake was considered a major undertaking.[37]

The importance of knowing that someone cared was magnified for those who didn't have visitors. Some people there did not even have family support. One nurse remembered that the family of one young man and his father never visited them. After the two died, she found an unsent letter among the younger man's belongings. One of the lines read, "Don't think tuberculosis killed me. I died because nobody cared."[38]

All of the entertainments and activities surely helped to pass the time, but their true importance may have been the opportunity for patients to hold on to a sense of normalcy. Even though confined to bed, they were informed of world news and were encouraged to keep in touch with friends and families. They celebrated holidays, watched movies, and played pranks on fellow patients.

Dr. Mariette's strategies had an impact. A World War I veteran wrote in a letter to his mother, "The superintendent wants everyone in the San to have a good time. I guess they think contentment has something to do with recovery from the way they act." That meant the staff, too, he said, because someone told his doctor that "happy nurses mean happy patients."[39]

11

Tuberculosis and Children

THE CONTENTMENT STRATEGY ALSO EXTENDED to younger patients at the Children's Building. About fifty children lived there at any one time. Most of them were not particularly ill, but had what was called "childhood tuberculosis" or "first infection." The purpose of their stay was to prevent development of active TB. Some children had bone TB, which was not contagious but required braces and casts to prevent deformities.

The building was designed with a bay window jutting out into the balcony, so a nurse sitting there would be able to watch children in two wards and the balcony at once. Babies and children under five years old lived on the third floor, in two wards of five beds each. The nursery doors were locked, and no visitors were allowed in at any time. Relatives could see the babies through the windows of the nursery.[1]

That floor also had a balcony for sun treatment and four isolation rooms, where new arrivals were quarantined during the period of their first examinations. For a young child away from the familiar setting of home and family, it was a traumatic experience. The director of nurses, Jeanette Stenseth, acknowledged the loneliness of the newly admitted child who finds he must stay in a room by himself for several days. The isolation was necessary to protect all of the children from any infectious childhood diseases the new child might carry.[2]

Those isolation rooms loomed large in the memories of people who came to the sanatorium as children. LuDean Harmsen Pontius recalled her experience:

I was put on the third floor in an end room for quarantine for six weeks. . . . I was very unhappy when I first came here. I can remember them putting me in the bathtub and scrubbing me and

washing my hair, and I screamed the whole time. Then they cart-
ed me into this room. The kids talked to me, and then finally I
was able to get out and mingle with the kids. I think that six weeks
was probably pretty traumatic because I can remember a lot of
things. I wasn't really happy then.[3]

Susan Oss's memory of her first day is also vivid. She writes, "The first
day there I was put in a gray institutional steel crib in a small room by my-
self. I received my first dress-a-doll that day. She was beautiful, made of soft
rubber and wearing a blue voile dress. But I cried so hard that I threw up all
over the doll."[4]

Nurse Stenseth asserted that the tears disappeared once they joined the
other children and the fun began.[5] This was not an entirely false claim. The
staff tried to make the Children's Building a "happy place for each child who
must be separated from his family."[6]

The children shared pets, which at various times included a pony, dogs,
cats, chickens, goldfish, and chameleons. The pony was an unusual arrival,
which was reported by Wallace Erickson, age twelve:

This morning when we were playing ball the nurse came down
and said Dr. Hutchinson had a surprise for us. We thought it was
a dog at first, but when we came up to the car in the back seat was
a pony. She had won it at the Shiners' donkey baseball game. Its
name is Hutchy. We all like it very much.[7]

The school consisted of three teachers and a playground supervisor.
The students had the same course of study as other school children, and
they took the Stanford Achievement and Kuhlman-Anderson Intelligence
tests. Most students who returned to their regular schools were able to fit
in at the appropriate grade level. Children made deaf by tuberculosis were
given training in lip reading in addition to their schoolwork. Teachers took
turns working on Saturday and Sunday afternoons in order to discuss the
children's progress with parents during visiting hours.[8]

Children, especially only children, sometimes had difficulties adjusting
to life with so many other children. In these instances, the staff held what
they called an "adjustment conference." The conference was attended by the

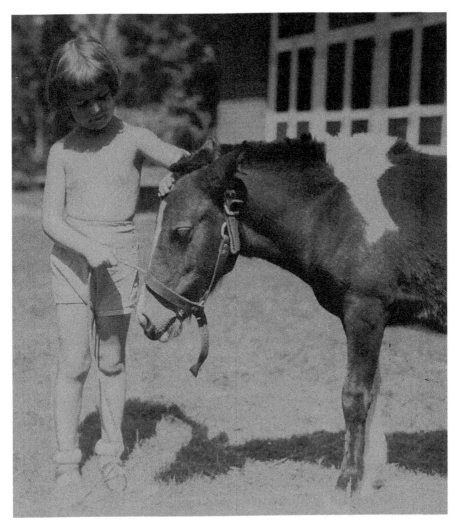

Pony donated by a doctor. (Courtesy of the Minnesota Historical Society)

child's social worker, physician, nurse, and teacher, all of whom reported their experiences with the child and created a plan to help ease the transition.[9]

Visitors were rarely allowed inside the Children's Building. All parents who were patients had to meet their children in the auditorium under strict restrictions. They could not touch or kiss, and had to maintain a distance while conversing.[10] Patients on exercise who had negative sputum could obtain permission from their doctor to walk with their children on the sanatorium grounds during warm months.[11]

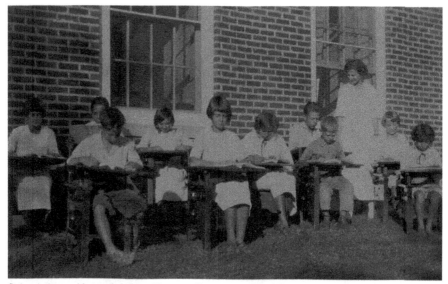

School class with teacher Mrs. Hauger. (Courtesy of the Minnesota Historical Society)

Some visitors were allowed to interact with children who did not have active tuberculosis. The baseball players from the Minneapolis Millers were especially well received when they arrived with bats and balls.

Day trips brought the children to local farms and towns, which they described in a monthly newsletter. "We went for a ride to Shakopee by the Minnesota River. We saw muskrat houses. We saw flocks of birds. We stopped to buy a honeycomb. We saw some pussy tails," reported Frederick Gallagher, age nine.[12]

Shakopee, about ten miles from Glen Lake, seems to have been a favorite destination for road trips:

Mrs. Hauger took the sixth, seventh, and ninth graders to Shakopee Springs. On our way there, we saw a little humble shack with a few garbage cans and goats along the hillside. I was very depressed at the looks of it. As we went on, we met the man who owned the house. We found that he lived all alone. When we reached the springs, we got out of the car and had some nice spring water. I surely enjoyed our ride.[13]

Also popular was the Brown Goat Farm, south of Hopkins. There the farmer, Ernest Matti, used the goat milk to make *gjetost* (brown Norwegian cheese) or Swiss cheese.[14]

The children were encouraged to have hobbies, keep scrapbooks, and make collections. Reading was highly encouraged, and so was listening to the radio or records. Girls who were old enough to sew could make their own dresses.

In the 1920s, in keeping with the heliotherapy treatment of the time, the children, stripped down to the waist, played out in the snow wearing not much more than loincloths, stockings, and boots.[15] An article in the *Minneapolis Journal* said, "The sight of naked children tobogganing down the slopes at Glen Lake in winter makes an adult, wrapped in heavy clothing, shiver."[16]

Dolores Romatko Farr remembered it as part of the therapy at the time, and they just took it for granted that they would go out. They thought every child did that. Delores was a poster child for the promotion of Christmas seals in 1938 and 1939. They made her take off her dress for photographs, to illustrate the sun therapy, but as a little girl she didn't appreciate having to do that in front of strangers.[17]

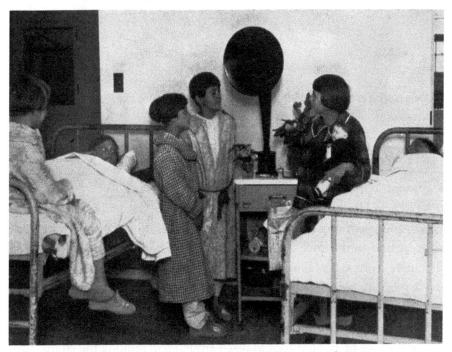

Children listening to a radio with an amplifier. (Courtesy of the Lokke Collection)

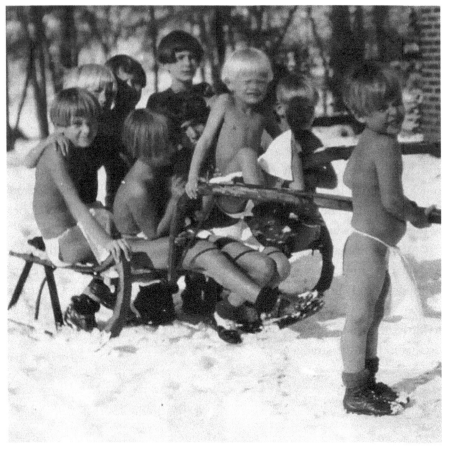

Children playing in the snow in loin cloths. (Courtesy of the Minnesota Historical Society)

The children also experienced surgeries and other medical interventions as needed. A variety of tractions, splints, and casts were used to immobilize joints and support bodies so healing could be achieved.

LuDean Harmsen had tuberculosis in her hips. She had quite a few surgeries, and spent most of her stay in a body cast down to the toes of her right leg and to the knee of the left one. A rod between her legs was used by nurses to raise and lower her body for bedpan use. LuDean admits she was a problem patient, and she would get out of bed and try to walk in the cast. Finally, after breaking a couple of casts, she was restrained in bed by a custom-made straitjacket that covered the entire bed. Even so, she was able to use the toes of her left foot to reach around and unhook the straps.

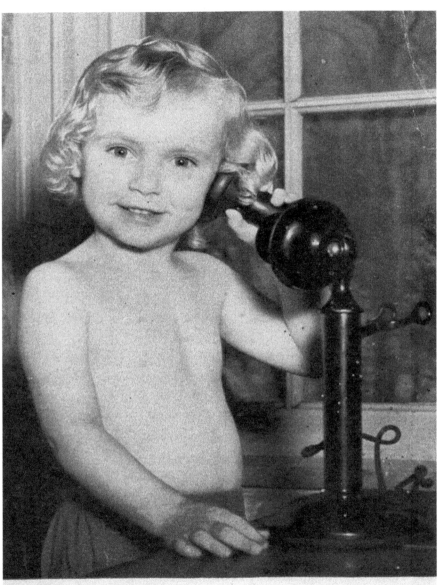

" I'm Line "
she says —

Dolores on a Christmas Seal postcard. (Author's collection)

In spite of the surgeries, the infection kept growing. Finally, they performed a final surgery, leaving a big window in the cast to expose the incision. There were no antibiotics in the 1930s, so the nurses treated the incision with silver nitrate. Eventually, the incision closed up and healed, and the tuberculosis was gone. After her eight-year stay in the Children's Building, everyone regarded it as a miracle.[18]

Gloria Yberra was eleven months old when she was brought to the sanatorium from General Hospital. She had both tuberculosis of the spine and contagious childhood pulmonary tuberculosis, which meant that she spent a few months in the main building before she arrived at the Children's Building. To prevent the TB from deforming her spine, she was strapped to a Bradford frame when she was four years old. For five years, she was on this stretcher-like bed with no springs or mattress. She ate, studied lessons, and played with her friend, June, who was similarly restrained. They did everything without leaving the frame. At age nine, Gloria was fitted with a brace to support her back, and she had to learn how to walk for the first time. She mastered walking and wore the brace for two years.[19]

One could assume that a discharge from the Children's Building would be regarded as a happy thing, but Gloria Stromseth wrote, "many children from deprived or difficult homes hated to leave Glen Lake and return to their old lives." She described her life there as almost idyllic, but admitted that having come to Glen Lake as a one-year-old, she had no memories of a previous home to compare it to.[20]

Dolores Romatko said she'd had a happy childhood. "It was like a family," she said. She saw the same nurses every day, and there was continuity.[21]

One young girl was in the Children's Building for a while before eventually going home to her parents. She was accustomed to having nurses on rotating shifts each day. She became impatient with her mother and said to her, "How come you are on duty all of the time?"[22]

LuDean Harmsen, who cried when she came, also cried when she left. "You're taking me away from my home," she told the social worker. "I really cried. That was a sad day. It was worse than when I came. It really was, because this was home."[23]

There was another group of children to be kept happy on the Glen Lake campus. It may have been a lesser challenge, because those who attended the summer camp near Birch Island Lake had fewer rules and more liberty.

Fresh-air camps opened in Minnesota after the turn of the century, following a model established on the East Coast. Ramsey County's summer camp for tuberculous children began operation in 1908 at Cherokee Heights in St. Paul on a bluff above the Mississippi River. The camp's medical director, Dr. Taylor, persuaded clubwomen to have Tag Day sales to raise money for the camp. For a small sum of money, a person could buy a printed paper tag and pin it to their dress or suit lapel. A sale in 1910 raised nearly $23,000 dollars, which subsidized the opening of the Eva Shapiro Memorial Camp at White Bear Lake, which was run by the Anti-Tuberculosis Committee.[24]

Minneapolis's first summer camp for children was established by the Christian family in 1906. Two years later, the Visiting Nurses Committee opened a new summer camp at Riverside Park on Eighth Street South. In 1909, the Visiting Nurses Committee tent camp moved to Glenwood Park (later renamed Theodore Wirth Park). In 1925, the Visiting Nurses summer camp moved to the Glen Lake Sanatorium campus, where the Citizens' Aid Society built permanent structures. The camp's location was south of the

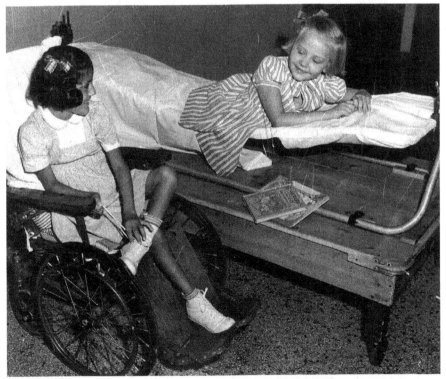

Gloria (tying her shoes) and June on frame. (Courtesy of the Hennepin History Museum)

main building and west of the power plant, near the shore of Birch Island Lake.[25]

The Glen Lake camp served about fifty children, who ranged in age from three to sixteen years old. It was usually open from the first Monday after school closed in June until the last week in August. The children were expected to understand that the camp was not a vacation home but a place where work and play, food and rest, and all other activities were focused on health building.[26]

Irv Hanson worked as a summer camp counselor in 1927, and he later described the boys he was charged with as a "motley crew," from indigent parentage, thin, bedraggled, and pitiful. Some, he said, had ribs like xylophones. His job was to take care of the boys, and also to be the lifeguard at Excelsior Beach when the children went swimming. Hanson's wages were thirty dollars every two weeks plus board, which included a tent for living quarters.

He supervised competitions in athletic events, such as free throws, punt and pass, and baseball. Each boy won a prize of some type, and Hanson used his Wednesdays off to make a trip to Dayton's Department Store to find numerous cheap prizes (and also to see the Minneapolis Millers play if they were in town). Hanson was surprised by the boys' desire to read, and he made sure that library books were provided for them. As the summer neared its end, the ribs were no longer evident, and he reported that the boys were tearful and sad at leaving.[27]

The success of the summer camps was noted by the *Northwestern Health Journal*, which cited the Glen Lake camp and one established by St. Louis County Public Health Association at Prairie Lake, about fifty miles from Duluth. Both camps received financial assistance from Christmas seals as part of tuberculosis prevention activity. The journal article called the summer outings a "Road to Health" that provided lasting lessons in correct living.[28]

Most of the campers at Glen Lake were recommended by Minneapolis public school nurses. The children had regular visits from a physician, usually doctors Fenger, Mattill, or Hutchinson. They had tuberculin and blood tests, X-rays, vision tests, and dental work. The administrators of the summer camp program intended to send the children back to their homes healthier and happier in all ways possible.[29]

The summer camp children lived in a long dormitory, with a wing for boys and another for girls. Rooms for some of the counselors were in the center. The recreation hall and dining room were combined in another building.[30] The children ate meals delivered from the sanatorium kitchen. The children could drink as much milk and eat as many helpings of food as they wanted.[31]

The day's activities began at 6:45 a.m. with flag ceremonies. During the day the children would sunbathe, do handicrafts, rest, swim, and have both planned and unsupervised play. At night the campers listened to stories, and knelt by their beds and recited the Lord's Prayer in unison. Lights were turned off at 9:15 p.m. They had a non-sectarian Sunday school, an occasional Mass or visit from a rabbi, movies on Wednesday nights, and picnics on Thursday nights.[32]

Because of age differences, the camp staff provided three programs. Small children were kept occupied with puppies, a sandbox, playground equipment, and toys. The older children played softball and volleyball, went on overnight hikes, and fished.[33] Older girls at the camp had a sewing circle under the trees, and Boy Scouts continued their activities at the camp with a volunteer scoutmaster.[34] Both genders learned archery.

Parents came to the camp to visit their children on Saturday and Sunday afternoons. If the child's parent was a patient, visiting was limited to twice a month in the auditorium. Because neither group had active tuberculosis, the Children's Building and summer camp children would have picnics and softball games together.

The lake on which the camp stood was more like a marsh and not suitable for swimming, so the children traveled to nearby Lake Minnetonka in a large truck. Angeline Wanecki, age twelve, was enthusiastic about the excursions to a beach near the city of Excelsior. "We go swimming four times a week: Tuesday, Thursday, Friday, and Saturday. About thirty-five children go each time. George takes us to Lake Minnetonka in the truck. When George gets a sudden streak of ambition, he takes us on the roller coaster road. Then's the time we hold our breaths!"[35] The roller coaster road to which Angeline referred is Williston Road in Minnetonka between Excelsior Boulevard and Highway 7. Originally very hilly, it was subdued by reconstruction in the 1990s.

Mrs. George C. Christian, daughter-in-law of George H. and Lenore Hall Christian, continued the family's interest in the children's welfare. Each Fourth of July she visited to personally provide flags, horns, caps, and bal-

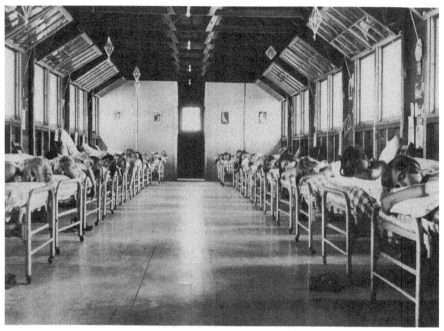

Summer camp dormitory. (Courtesy of the Minnesota Historical Society)

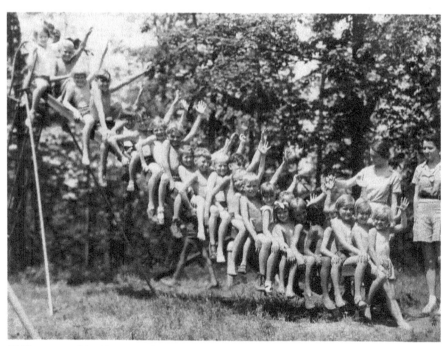

Children on a slide. (Courtesy of the Minnesota Historical Society)

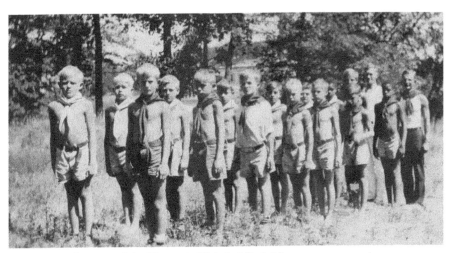

Boy Scouts. (Courtesy of the Minnesota Historical Society)

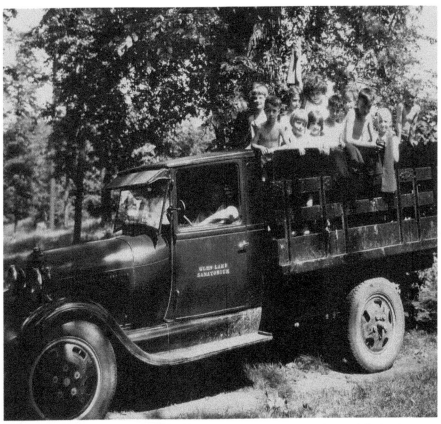

Truck used to take children swimming. (Courtesy of the Minnesota Historical Society)

loons for a party. Sometimes she led the children in a march around the camp and then visited with each child individually before she left.[36]

Parents who had children at the camp were asked for their opinions of the experience. Some of their responses indicated:

* The children learn to live with others and learn to be more thoughtful.
* Their appreciation of beauty and cleanliness has been increased.
* They go back to their homes with more self-reliance and self-confidence.
* Habits of punctuality are formed.
* They show improvement in school.
* They have many new interests.

Not all children appreciated being there, as indicated by the camp director's report:

It is a curious commentary on child life of today that not many boys over twelve years of age are contented and happy there, while the girls are. At home, the boys have their "gang life," they

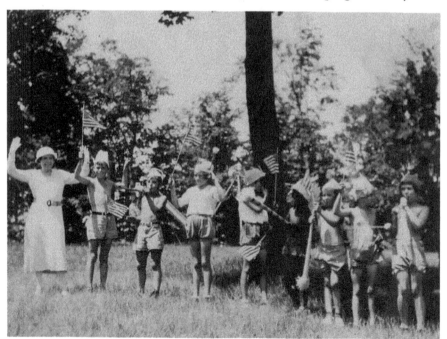

Mrs. Christian. (Lunde scrapbook. Courtesy of the Minnesota Historical Society)

go swimming, to the movies and stay out late at night without much apparent restriction. So life at Camp seems tame to them. For that reason we are limiting the Camp to younger children and leaving the older boys to seek their camp life elsewhere.[37]

Irv Hanson's description of indigent children might well have been accurate at that point of the Great Depression, but members of the Leaf family, who were there in the mid-1930s, remember a different sort of camper. Their father had a steady job working for the Milwaukee Railroad. Their large garden put plenty of good food on the table, but the family did not have the money to pay for four children to spend a summer at camp.

Their paternal grandmother had lived with them and was diagnosed with advanced tuberculosis in 1932, shortly before her death. In view of Mrs. Leaf's close contact with TB, and her continuing daily tasks of running a household with four children, a public health nurse recommended that the three older children—Earl, Lorraine, and Delbert—go to summer camp at Glen Lake Sanitorium. This served a dual purpose of building up resistance in the children and giving their mother some needed respite. The children spent three summers at the camp, joined in 1935 by their little sister, Carol.

While at the camp, they wore few clothes to have as much exposure to the sun and fresh air as possible. Boys wore shorts, and girls wore shorts and halter tops, or no above-waist covering at all if they were very young. The children would lie in the sun, first on their backs to get sun on their chests, and then they would turn over to get sun on their backs. While lying there a counselor read to them from a book, which was continued from day to day.

At the end of the summer a prize was given to the girl and boy who had the best suntans. The person who judged the suntans would pull down the elastic waist of the children's shorts to expose the light area which shorts covered. The greatest contrast between that area and the tanned area above it would determine the winner. Lorraine had very white skin but tanned easily, and one year she won the prize.

In 1935, two other families had four children each at the camp: the Breedloves of North Minneapolis and the Cupkas of Minneapolis. The Breedloves were the only black children at the camp. Their mother came to the camp each Sunday to wash daughter Josephine's hair and then braid it into a hairdo that lasted until the next Sunday.

Lorraine Leaf recalled that those summers were a wonderful respite for her mom and dad. "It must have been like a second honeymoon for them, especially that third summer when my sister was also with us at camp and they could enjoy life as a couple again." A baby brother was born the following May.[38]

As with the older patients and their contemporaries in the Children's Building, the young campers benefitted from Dr. Mariette's philosophy of treating the whole person, not just the disease. Whether they were contented or not, though, all patients looked forward to the day they would be discharged. And for every effort at contentment, there were several reasons to not be contented.

12

The Not-So-Good Roaring '20s

IN SPITE OF EFFORTS BY DR. MARIETTE and his staff to keep the patients contented, not everyone was. People could be uncomfortable in a culture that strove for normalcy and that also put great emphasis on cheerfulness, even if forced. One anonymous author compared Glen Lake to the army:

> Arrange everything at home so you can be gone for a time which depends on the duration of the war, then you go to camp where you start training. Your ordinary clothes are taken away, someone tells you where you are to sleep and you suddenly find yourself lost in a bewildering set of rules, which seem to cover all the activities of life. Much of the liberty of adult life must be given up, when to get up and when to go to bed, what you eat and when, are all decided for you. You are not only expected to obey all rules but you are told to be cheerful about it.[1]

There were so many things associated with a normal life that the patients couldn't do. For Judy Smykal, who had pulmonary tuberculosis and couldn't go outside, a main memory of her time at the sanitorium was the loss of the sky. She was always inside a structure. When she was finally allowed to go home on leave, it was almost overwhelming to see the sky again because it had been withheld for so long.[2]

Most patients understood that a particular activity was prohibited because of the adverse effect it could have on healing and a successful recovery. Understanding it didn't mean they didn't resent it, though. That was especially true of two prohibitions that involved addictive habits: smoking and drinking.

The sanatorium's rules on smoking need to be understood within the context of the era. Studies linking cigarette smoking to cancer wouldn't be published until the 1950s, so the smoking ban was not based on health issues. The physicians attempted to keep patients from smoking for two reasons:

(1) improperly discarded cigarette butts could spread tuberculosis, and
(2) patients smoking in bed could burn the place down.[3]

Indeed, many of the doctors at Glen Lake were themselves smokers. One of them supported a ban on cigarettes only because smoking increased patients' pulse and circulation, which he thought might promote an exchange between the body's organs and spread the tuberculosis infection.[4] A smoking policy in the 1920s simply stated the institution could not prevent smoking, but discouraged it.[5] However, in order to set a good example, medical staff and other employees were requested to refrain from smoking in front of the patients.[6]

The other banned substance, liquor, was not much of a problem when the sanatorium opened. The Eighteenth Amendment to the U.S. Constitution, the Volstead Act, established nationwide prohibition in 1920, when Glen Lake was only four years old.

In the 1920s, admission to sanatoriums in Minnesota was still mostly voluntary. Under the 1913 sanatorium law, cities that had public health officers could declare a person a public health menace if he or she had positive tuberculosis and was endangering the health of others. This included working with food after having been told not to do so, spitting in public, or exposing family members to the disease. In those cases, the law stated that the public health officer had the power to remove the offending persons and place them in a hospital or sanatorium, upon approval by the county commissioners. That sometimes meant authorizing a sheriff to escort the offender to the institution if they wouldn't go willingly.[7]

In reality, it was extremely difficult for an institution that was essentially a hospital to physically restrain a patient. A sheriff could deliver him to a sanatorium, but in several cases, the patient left immediately and "beat the sheriff home." Guards cost money, and limited budgets prevented sanatoriums from hiring them.[8]

Glen Lake also received people who either acquired tuberculosis in one of the state's mental hospitals or were not accepted at a state hospital because of pre-existing TB. In 1925, sanatorium staff requested to have "one room in each wing fitted with a heavy mesh screen for irrational patients."[9] In 1928, there was a need to procure "some sort of straight jacket or other restraint for insane patients at the Sanatorium."[10] Many requests to the legislature to fund alternative, secure housing for incorrigible or out-of-control tuberculous patients fell on deaf ears.

Other habits and activities were addressed through specific policies. Spitting, or expectorating, could bring disciplinary action. Posted notices told patients they were prohibited from expectorating in the wash bowls and on the ground, and that doing so could be reason for expulsion. Patients were reminded also to observe public health cautions about kissing and licking postage stamps. They were told to drink milk out of glasses, not milk bottles. One patient who was careless about his sputum was no longer allowed to eat in the dining room but was put on bedside tray service.[11]

Even relatively harmless pastimes came under scrutiny. Card-playing was a favorite activity for many patients, but strict religious norms of the 1920s meant that patients couldn't play cards in the auditorium or any other public place on Sunday, a rule that also included playing pool.[12] Any form of gambling was especially prohibited, but small-time wagering existed anyway. Poker-playing patients caused recurring problems when cheating led to arguments.

Patients were also not allowed to be in specific parts of the main building. Those had been declared "clean" areas for the staff and visitors, as opposed to the patient areas, which were considered contaminated. Included on the clean list and, thus, off-limits were the nurses' desks, medicine rooms, the front lobby, the visitors' lounge on Main West, and telephones in those areas.[13]

Patients had to accept a lack of privacy as the norm. Almost all lived in wards, with their personal spaces separated only by bedside tables and very rarely by curtains. Patients heard others coughing and making sniffling sounds.[14] Patients who had to wash themselves or change clothes in bed did it awkwardly under a blanket for privacy. Everyone disliked using the metal bedpans in winter. One patient recalled using one out on the porch, while trying to keep warm under the covers. "It was terrible," she said, noting that warmer summer weather wasn't much better because it made odors more noticeable.[15]

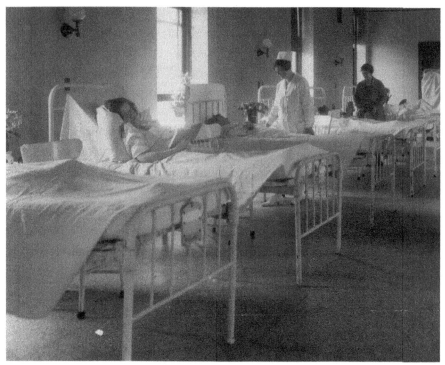

No privacy curtains. (Courtesy of the Lokke Collection)

The lack of central heating and air conditioning also contributed to discontent. With radiator heat, there was no flow of circulated air. Windows remained ajar in all but the worst winter weather to provide fresh air. During summer heat waves, the propeller-shaped cage fans oscillated slowly and hummed loudly.

Even the caregivers could be a source of irritation. Nurses bustled in and out of rooms attending to patients who required frequent dressing changes or had episodes of high fevers and restlessness. A good nurse could promote contentment, but a sadistic one could make life miserable. Some who enjoyed wielding power responded slowly to requests or "forgot" to wash a patient's hair. Strict bed patients were especially vulnerable and feared retribution if they complained.

Not all ministerial visits were of help to the patients, either. One pastor was overheard telling a teenager that he should spend his time at the sanatorium contemplating his sins. The same clergyman also refused to speak at a service because the sanatorium auditorium was unsanctified.[16]

The relative isolation of the sanatorium was exacerbated during winter months by frequent quarantines in response to epidemics raging in the outside world. In 1928, an especially bad year for colds and strep throat, visitors were excluded and leaves were cancelled from December 17 until January 14 of 1929, in spite of the Christmas holiday. The Shriners were able to come to the sanatorium to host their annual party on December 22, but that was countered by the announcement that no patients could go to the Shrine Circus on January 21.[17]

Sometimes the discontent was generated by people who were not compatible being trapped in a ward together. A continuing disturbance on Main East in a ward of six patients was traced to one man who made himself a nuisance. He was transferred into a single room on the same floor. Although that resulted in a harmonious ward for the remaining patients, it became evident that moving to a single room was regarded as a reward for misbehaving patients. The medical staff then decided that "those with habits that rendered them undesirable roommates should not be allowed to tie up single rooms to the detriment of sick patients but rather grouped into one ward." The alternative would be to leave the institution.[18]

Although one of the missions of the sanatorium was to isolate the tuberculous person from the general population, there were times when uncooperative patients were discharged. People were given many opportunities to mend their ways. One man left and was readmitted thirteen times. In the years in which waiting lists existed, though, it seemed wasteful to cater to malcontents when other people needed help.[19]

Quite possibly the least normal and most aggravating situation in the sanatorium was the segregation of the genders. Romances were discouraged and sexual liaisons prohibited. There wasn't any sermonizing about immorality, because the main concern, as with smoking, was health related. Sexual intercourse is strenuous exercise that raises one's heart rate and respiration, and, thus, could be harmful for someone with pulmonary tuberculosis.

Patients still flirted and the sanatorium version of dating served as ways to attain normalcy and distance themselves from their illness. Pairing off was prohibited by the medical staff, even for married couples, and prompted disciplinary action if discovered. The sanatorium tried to rely on "good sense and good breeding" to guide individual behavior, but patients were not allowed to go walking with other patients or employees of the opposite sex.

Mixed-gender activity was officially limited to chaperoned social times in the auditorium or dining room.

Living in the Shadow of Death describes "cousining" as a term used in sanatoriums to describe relationships, especially those between\people who were married, but not to each other. The term's popularity may have been limited. It does not appear in Glen Lake documents or in writing or interviews with patients.[20]

The tunnels, on the other hand, loom large in the writings and memories of patients. It is hard to imagine a less romantic spot than a damp concrete burrow, but 2,500 feet of tunnels offered several nooks and crannies for couples. The secluded passageways also transported water, electricity, and steam to the buildings through overhead pipes. The occasional leaks were tolerated, and no one knew they had reason to be concerned about the asbestos insulation.

In 1929, a posted notice banned male East Cottage patients from escorting female patients through the tunnel to their West Cottage.[21] One clever patient added graffiti to the sign that pointed to the cottages: "East Cottage + West Cottage = Children's Building."[22]

Dora Cohen, dietician, remembered that the tunnels were quite a scene. "Sometimes it was difficult to walk by. It was understandable—they were young people, and they were confined to their rooms for months at a time."[23] Lois Johnson remembers visiting her husband, Howard. "We'd go out and eat in the hall or sometimes even down in the tunnels just to be by ourselves."[24]

Patients became acquainted with each other during the work-up portion of privileges, when they could leave their room in litters or wheelchairs. Some staff members were sympathetic to the patients' need to seek and receive affection. Patients offered bribes to bed pushers and orderlies in order to get placed next to each other at the Wednesday movie nights and cuddle a bit while the auditorium was dark. The lines that formed for the weighing room and pneumothorax treatments were also welcomed opportunities for flirting.

With limited opportunities for face-to-face meetings, though, patients got creative. Men and women from the east and west wings communicated with flashlights at night or mirrors during the day. Morse code was used, but too many patients learned it, so couples devised their own codes for certain phrases.

Sometimes ambulatory patients or orderlies delivered notes and messages to people in other wards, but resourceful methods of communication were also devised. Patients wrote messages on pieces of fruit or balls and tossed them from one bed to another.[25] One nurse remembers seeing oranges roll down the hallway between the east and west wings. Passersby kicked them along to their destination.[26]

Rules that prohibited "pairing off" met with mixed success. If a couple was determined to consummate a relationship, there were places less public than the tunnel. Frederick Manfred was amused that the doctors couldn't figure out how a woman on One West became pregnant. He said that patients were well aware of when the linen closets would not be in use.[27]

It's a testament to the power of love over rules that several patients married after their discharge. It is also a reflection of a change in attitude that once held sway when tuberculosis was thought to be hereditary. Dr. Bell stated an opinion held by many when he told the State Medical Association in 1897 that intermarriage of consumptives should be made "odious by every possible means." He suggested the possibility of legislation prohibiting marriage "among this particular class of people."[28]

During Evelyn Roland's stay at Glen Lake, she met the Reverend Milton Wolter, also a patient. Many people thought it was risky for two tuberculous people to marry, but they did anyway. The couple later ministered at churches in Minnesota, California, and Illinois. Her husband died in 1994 and she died in 2002, at the age of ninety.[29]

Employees also formed romantic attachments. Dr. Funk's future wife, Myrtle, was a nurse when he started work in 1924 as a junior intern. In 1925, she was diagnosed with active TB and went on the cure. She wasn't discharged until Christmas 1928 and they married in January.[30]

A few employees gave cause for concern because of their social activities in those pre-penicillin days. The 1928 medical staff meeting minutes emphasized that was against the law for employees with communicable diseases to work in kitchens. If employees did not pay their bills for treatment of venereal diseases, their wages could be garnished.[31]

By the 1920s most medical professionals acknowledged that tuberculosis blossomed in families because of the close quarters of habitation. At that time, many homes in rural Hennepin County still lacked indoor plumbing and water for bathing and laundry. City water and sewer infrastructure

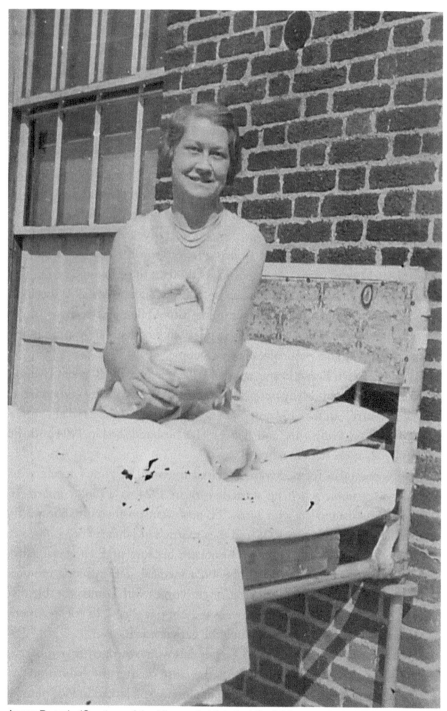

Agnes Dvorak. (Courtesy of the Minnesota Historical Society)

had yet to reach many homes even in Minneapolis. Outhouses, cisterns, and wells were still the norm for some families and not necessarily as a result of poverty.

Agnes Dvorak was twenty-five years old in 1923 and a patient at Glen Lake when her mother died from TB at Clear Springs in present-day Minnetonka. Agnes, a patient off and on for eleven and a half years, was engaged to marry a fellow patient, but she contracted meningitis and died in 1930. Her fiancé, Oscar, was also a patient, and he remained at Glen Lake as a bookkeeper.[32]

Henry Earl Partridge entered Ah-gwah-ching Sanatorium, while his wife Myrtle lived in a boarding house in Minneapolis and worked as an elevator operator in a hospital. Their daughter, born in 1926, lived with her maternal grandparents in northern Minnesota. Henry died in 1931. Myrtle also contracted TB and died in 1933 at Glen Lake.[33]

For parents entering the sanatorium, separation from family was heartbreaking.

Adele Boquist Oberg recalled her experience:

The bottom dropped out when I heard the verdict that I had TB. . . . Six weeks later my second little girl was born. I'll never forget the day I left home. My little boy, five, and little girl, three, ran along the boulevard waving "good-bye" to me. The baby of four months, whom I had never taken care of, was with us going to the Children's Building. I wondered if I would ever come back. . . . My babe was almost three when I took care of her for the first time. For three years I had not been inside my home.[34]

In 1929, two female patients about to be discharged were judged by courts to be unable to care for their families. For one, the medical staff agreed that her children be sent elsewhere when she went home. The other woman was summoned to appear regarding the adoption of her children, including one born at the sanatorium. The social services department was asked to intervene in this case, and later census records indicate that the family did remain intact.[35]

Few avenues of intimacy existed for parents, whose physical contact with their children was not only discouraged, but actively prevented. Children under the age of sixteen were not allowed into the main building except to the auditorium on Saturdays. Infants and very young children were to be left at home. Families stood on the lawn under their relative's window and exchanged waves and blown kisses. Patients with children could obtain permission to be wheeled to the auditorium for Saturday visiting hours, but there were restrictions. Children could not be hugged or touched but had to stay six feet away from their parents.

Some women gave birth during their stay at the sanatorium. A few doctors believed that pregnancy would not affect a woman's tuberculosis or could even be beneficial if the growing fetus acted as a crutch for the lungs. Others thought the extra work load on all organs wasn't worth the risk. Doctors at Glen Lake recommended therapeutic abortions in some cases when the mother's life was clearly endangered.

When a birth did occur, every precaution was taken to prevent the baby's contact with anyone who might have tuberculosis. The nurse receiving the baby had to avoid contact with the mother, other patients, or anything that might have been handled by patients. Babies were immediately removed from the birthing room and taken to the nursery in the nearby Children's Building.[36]

Occasionally a newborn showed signs of the disease and then was kept in the main building, so as to not expose other children to active tuberculosis. A sanatorium mother was not allowed to even see her child until it was six weeks old and then could not hold the baby but had to look at it from six feet away. Subsequent visiting depended on a doctor's permission.[37]

In spite of those restrictions, several pregnant ex-patients asked to be readmitted to the sanatorium to have their babies, because they felt more comfortable having an obstetrician who was familiar with their history of tuberculosis.[38]

Adjusting to sanatorium life was difficult for anyone who became a patient, but it might have been especially challenging for those who were not white. In general, the few non-white patients who were at Glen Lake during the 1920s are invisible except in the statistical records. Their history with tuberculosis is significant, because of an early twentieth-century tie between the social philosophy of eugenics and the neglect or sterilization of people considered to be unfit. In a 1911 book, *Heredity in Relation to Eugenics*, Charles Davenport claimed that only the "submerged tenth" of the population was susceptible to tuberculosis. Eugenicists insisted that "unfit" people died because of defective genes and not from germs.[39] Some eugenically minded doctors mixed their philosophies with the prejudices of the time and extended their definition of "unfit" to non-European or non-white ethnicities and races.

Physicians in the 1800s often named racial susceptibility as the reason why "whole families of Indians, Negroes, and Mexicans" were dying from tuberculosis. Even though Dr. Allen Krause of Johns Hopkins University deserves credit for discrediting that notion by rightly pointing to living con-

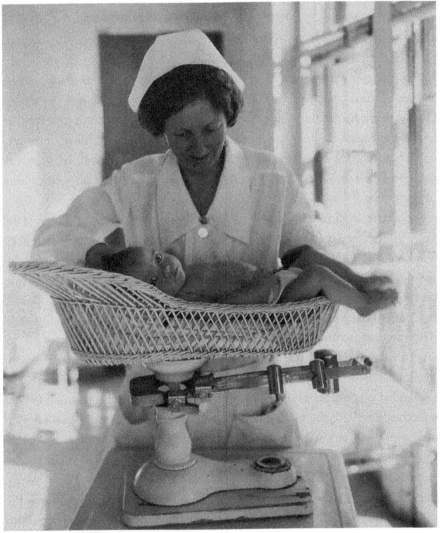

Baby being weighed. (Courtesy of the Minnesota Historical Society)

ditions, he perpetuated other harmful stereotypes by blaming those same groups for having the "common living habits of savages and semi-savages."[40]

Glen Lake treated very few Hispanic people in the 1920s. Migrant workers had arrived in Minnesota from Mexico early in the twentieth century to help with sugar beet harvests. They lived primarily in the Red River Valley and were served by Sunnyrest Sanatorium in Crookston. A small population residing in St. Paul used the Ramsey County facilities.

The black population at Glen Lake was never large. Only 100 patients of color were admitted from 1916 to 1933. Leon Nichols, the first black patient, died there in May of 1917. The U.S. census data for 1930 lists 701 patients at the sanatorium. Of those, seven were black, one of whom was a child. Only one of the seven was born in Minnesota. The others migrated from southern states. Among the employees that year, only one was black, and he was an elevator operator, a job often held by an ex-patient.

In Minneapolis, the death rate for African Americans with tuberculosis had always been higher than that for whites. In 1913, the death rate was 534.5 per 100,000 compared to 118 for the general population. In 1924, the rate had fallen to 303.6, but was still higher than the general population rate of sixty-nine.[41]

There is no definitive reason for the disparity, but one contributor is the lower economic status in which anyone who is sick feels compelled to keep working. Most of the black Americans worked at unskilled labor or in domestic positions. By waiting until their tuberculosis was far advanced before seeking medical help, their admission to a sanatorium was usually followed by death. That led to a high institutional death rate for blacks that would then discourage others from hospitalization.

In 1915, Booker T. Washington had initiated a national health movement that came to be known as Negro Health Week. The eight-day week began and ended on Sunday, in order to capitalize on communities' connections to churches. In 1926, the Hennepin County Tuberculosis Association cooperated with the Minneapolis Urban League for a special tuberculosis education campaign. In 1929, the observance of Negro Health Week coincided with an early diagnosis effort sponsored by the same association. St. Peter's Methodist church hosted guest speakers Dr. W.F. Grant from Cook County, Illinois, and Dr W.D. Brown from the Minneapolis Urban League. They urged attendees to participate in tuberculosis screening programs.[42]

Chapter sixteen in the book *Bargaining for Life* is titled "P.S. I am . . . Colored." Although it is primarily about Philadelphia, some of the comments about the reluctance for minority races to enter a sanatorium hold true for Glen Lake. Even where there weren't laws about segregation, blacks were reluctant to enter a mostly white facility and face racial insults or humiliation. Most sanatorium magazines published racist jokes, and *Terrace Topics* was no exception. The August 1935 issue said that one of the patients knew the "cutest story about two little negro babies" and those interested in hearing it would get a cordial welcome on Second West porch. The homecoming issue of September 1941 was less coy, relating an dialect joke about a black woman (considered racist by today's standards).

Patients from minority populations did not find a reflection in the medical or nursing staff at Glen Lake, which was almost entirely white up until the 1940s. In 1927, the medical staff discussed a letter from the University of Minnesota informing them that two "colored" interns were scheduled to come to the sanatorium. Staff responded to the Department of Medicine by telling them that the sanatorium had no objections if their classmates did not object to sleeping in the same room and eating with them.[43]

Also in 1927, a doctor was referred to Dr. Mariette for a position on the sanatorium staff. After some discussion, the medical staff decided that doctor's work was not "of sufficient high caliber (irrespective of color) to warrant his obtaining the position."[44]

It is unfortunate that Dr. Mariette's crusade for contented patients did not include an effort to make the sanatorium more welcoming for a specific population with a high rate of tuberculosis infection. He attributed the lowered death rates to isolation of contagious cases in a sanatorium, and that would have held true for black families as well as white.

African Americans in the state's sanatoriums probably fared better than Minnesota's Native American population. Up until 1924, when the Snyder Act of 1921 granted full citizenship to indigenous people, some counties argued that they and the state had no responsibility to accept American Indians into their sanatoriums. Until that year, there was also no facility in the state dedicated to the care of tuberculous Native Americans. Onigum Sanatorium opened in an unused federal school in 1924, which was seventeen years after the state sanatorium opened near the reservation. Prior to that, medical care was sporadic and delivered primarily by public health nurses.[45]

Glen Lake Sanatorium's distance from the reservations meant that its American Indian patients were few. The 1930 census for Glen Lake listed one female patient and two Native American nurses living on the campus. In 1946, when Inez contracted TB, she was admitted as a patient at Glen Lake because she lived with an aunt in Minneapolis. While there, she gave birth to fraternal twins at the sanatorium, and they were brought to a Catholic orphanage in St. Paul. The boy was eventually adopted into a white family.[46]

Native Americans came to the sanatorium mostly as entertainers, and on field trips to Shakopee by the children they seemed to serve the same purpose: "Mrs. Grenier took us on a ride yesterday to see the Indians. We saw some corn drying by an Indian house. An Indian squaw [sic] was washing some clothes."[47]

No matter what their race or economic or marital status, patients experienced the same roller coaster emotions of optimism and despair. They all hoped for a permanent cure. Their hopes were raised at the end of the 1920s, when British bacteriologist Sir Alexander Fleming noticed that green

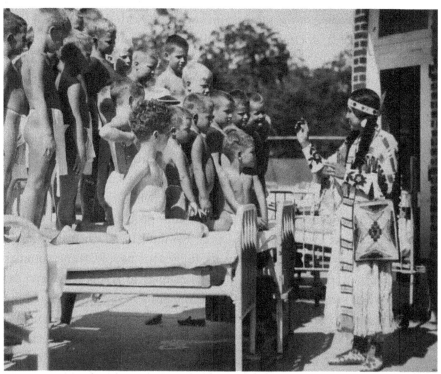

Indian entertainer. (Courtesy of the Minnesota Historical Society)

mold growing in a culture plate destroyed the bacteria around it. The mold, *Penicillin notatum*, was the first source of the penicillin antibiotic.[48] Although it was heralded as the cure for tuberculosis, it proved to be ineffective, and hopes were dashed.

In general, though, the decade of the 1920s was good to Glen Lake and its patients. The institution was well-funded by both the state legislature and Hennepin County. Dr. Mariette and the medical staff published several papers in medical journals, and Glen Lake received national recognition for its innovations and achievements.

In 1927, Glen Lake hired Charlotte Keyes, a statistician, and Frances Nemec, a registered nurse and registered records librarian. Together they established a medical records room. Nemec set up an index of diseases from the records of all past Glen Lake patients because no universal classification existed at that time. In that same year, Glen Lake became the first U.S. tuberculosis sanatorium accredited by the American College of Surgeons under hospital standards established in 1921.

The campus expansions had brought its capacity to more than 700 beds, three times the number of beds recommended as a standard in ratio to population. In spite of this, Glen Lake still had a waiting list in April 1927. There

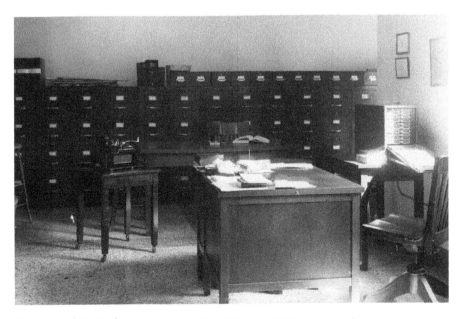

Medical records chart room. (Courtesy of the Hennepin History Museum)

were thirty-two far-advanced cases on the list, ten of whom were hospitalized at the Thomas Hospital for lack of space at the sanatorium.[49]

The commissioners voted to open an outpatient clinic at Glen Lake. The clinic served patients on the waiting list by providing pre-admission treatment and follow-up services. The sanatorium also operated clinics jointly with the University of Minnesota and the Hennepin County Tuberculosis Association. Clinic patrons were generally prospective sanatorium patients or ex-patients who couldn't afford the services of a regular physician. Physicians and nurses also called on patients who were receiving bed treatment in their own homes.

An article in *Minnesota Medicine* commented on the success of Glen Lake Sanatorium: "The institution proved popular, it was soon filled, a waiting list was created and, contrary to the usual custom, patients were apparently eager to enter the sanatorium."[50] Not only to enter, but to stay. The onset of the Great Depression meant that many patients on the road to better health considered themselves lucky to have a place to sleep and be well fed. The challenges that lay ahead in the 1930s would test the staff's ability to maintain the high standards and welcoming atmosphere they had worked so hard to attain.

13

Challenges in the 1930s

IN JANUARY 1930, GLEN LAKE SANATORIUM started its fifteenth year. It had matured from a small cottage-type sanatorium into an accredited hospital. The sanatorium's growing pains seemed to be over. Students from its medical and nursing school affiliates supplemented an established staff of physicians and nurses. Surgical procedures for the treatment of tuberculosis were still risky but generally regarded as an acceptable intervention.

As a form of celebration, Dr. Frank Jennings headed a committee that organized a homecoming for former patients in 1930. Perhaps it seems odd that patients who had left the sanatorium should feel loyalty to it. For many people, however, it had served as their home for more than two years. Good times and arguments and disappointments occurred in the sanatorium family, just like any other. Many friendships are forged in adversity, and the homecoming allowed friends to share memories. Their healthful presence also served to encourage the current patients and give them hope for recovery.

The first homecoming featured a band concert, speeches, and supper on the lawn. At the second homecoming in 1931, attendees toured a new facility. A wing funded by the Citizens' Aid Society in memory of Henry Hall Christian had extended the main building to the east. It would be the last structure added to the campus.[1]

The sanatorium was full to overflowing in 1931. It averaged a daily census of 696 patients, which was near its bed capacity. On some days they exceeded capacity, and recently admitted patients spent a day or two in bed in a hallway. East and west wing porches were converted to wards, and some rooms for two were remodeled to hold three. At the time, the average bed capacity of public sanatoriums in the United States was a little less than 150, making Glen Lake one of the largest.

The Great Depression initially had little effect on Glen Lake's operation. Minnesota's diversified economy held off a sharp rise in unemployment after the 1929 crash, but by 1930, the effects of economic collapse were reach-

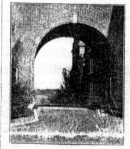

Homecoming Edition

TERRACE TOPICS

Vol. I No. 1   Oak Terrace, Minn. August 26, 1933   Price Five Cents

Greetings, Health Graduates!

WHAT'S GOING ON?

3:00 p.m. 'Step up and register!'
3:15   Music! Band concert in the Mall, with Knights Templar Band and Drill Team.
3:30   Visiting begins. Open house.
5:15   Supper. (You know where!)
7:00   An evening on the 'Streets of Paris'. Dancing; cigarette girls; the famed Louvre; Parisienne floor show; more dancing; refreshments!

Ceaseless Activity Marks Glen Lake's Fourth "Re-union"

Today is the big day—a red letter day. It's the day when nearly 100 ex-patients of Glen Lake Sanatorium and their families and friends gather once again at the scene of probably the biggest battle of their lives —the battle for health. These patients have won their fight against the insidious bug, and they are back to not only celebrate their victory, but to renew old acquaintances and help to cheer (by their presence) those of us who are still on the battlefield and who will soon be coming back ourselves to the same role.

Right at this minute there's commotion galore in "first corridor." It's crowded with "Health Graduates," laughing, talking and exchanging greetings. Typewriters are clicking away, "Step up and register," the typists call out. And how they step up! They're getting "labeled." (They're all marked men and women now!)

Registering through, they'll begin to saunter down the halls to greet familiar faces. Here's a fellow heading for 2nd East. I suppose that's his old floor. Another is taking the Main elevator, he is going way up to fourth or fifth, or will he call out "2nd" or "3rd"? There are a couple of girls wending their way west—and soon visitors will be flitting in and out of rooms on every floor. Talk about activity! This IS Homecoming!

Lots of patients get pleasant surprises. "Well, for heaven's sakes! Where have you been keeping yourself?" "Man, Joe, you're certainly looking swell." These are familiar phrases on this particular day—and rightly so.

Time goes so fast—TOO fast, and before you know it it's supper time. Have the

WELCOME!

Greetings

From Our

Superintendent

As superintendent, it is my great privilege, on behalf of the entire staff, to officially welcome you to Glen Lake Sanatorium today. The steady increase in attendance at the annual Homecomings is a matter of gratification to us and it is to you who have made these events so successful.

We are proud to use this magazine to cement that spirit of good will which is felt by the Sanatorium towards you and which you show that you reciprocate by your presence here. With kindest wishes for your future welfare, we welcome you back home.

Dr. E. S. Mariette

Alumni forgotten where the dining room is? Well I should say not! That line's the answer! Must feel like old times to them to eat cafeteria style up on "third." They haven't lost their appetites either—judging

Continued page 3

Annual Homecomings Become "Event of Year" to Glen Lake Alumni

F. L. JENNINGS M.D.

For weeks the 1933 Homecoming Committee has been looking forward to this year's event. We have planned it, worked out the details, overcome the obstacles, and it is the hope of the Committee that those attending the fourth Homecoming at Glen Lake Sanatorium will enjoy it as much as the Committee has enjoyed its part.

It seemed advisable to the Homecoming Committee of 1930 and to each succeeding Committee to have some form of entertainment, even though we fully realized that the visiting with old friends was the principle event of the day. At the first Homecoming in 1930, the entertainment consisted of a band concert, talks by several people interested in Glen Lake Sanatorium, and supper on the front lawn. At the 1931 Homecoming, the Citizens Aid Society of Minneapolis made the formal presentation to the Sanatorium of the new unit which gives such splendid quarters for our operating rooms, laboratory, and vocational training department. Last year the feature was a night club and this year we are inviting you to "The Streets of Paris."

It is a gratifying and encouraging sight to all now at the Sanatorium, patients, employes, and staff alike, to see the ex-patients return for Homecoming. There is a touch of pride that comes to those of us who have aided in a small way in the return to health of these "graduates." The idea of Homecoming had been considered by some of us for quite some time prior to 1930 because it was known that the idea had been successfully worked in other sanatoria. We now feel that the success of the Glen Lake Homecoming is well established and it has been decided that this shall be an annual event to be held on the last Saturday in August. An effort has been made each year to send notices to all ex-patients. This practice will be continued but I urge all to make a mental memorandum of this date so that no other plans will interfere with your returning each year.

The 1933 Homecoming edition of Terrace Topics. (Courtesy of the Minnesota Historical Society)

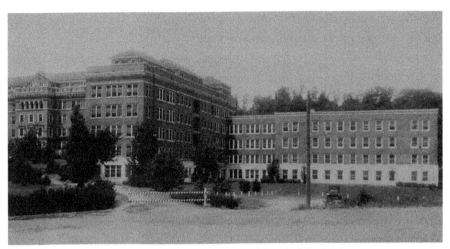

Completed east addition. (Courtesy of the Minnesota Historical Society)

ing the state.[2] In 1932, the sanatorium needed to achieve a two-percent cut in expenses, attempted primarily through reduction of food costs and waste.[3]

Glen Lake ran a relatively lean operation compared to other hospitals with similar functions. Its annual report for 1931 shows the daily cost of care per capita averaging $2.74 for three consecutive years, while the average cost in 1,100 general hospitals in the U.S. varied from $5.30 to $5.33. This did not go unnoticed by the American Hospital Association, which inspected the sanatorium.

> There is no institution that your inspector knows of in the United States giving professional and institutional care comparable to the service given at Glen Lake Sanatorium, and to so large a number of patients, that is being operated as economically as is Glen Lake Sanatorium or at a lesser total of operating disbursements. There may be institutions that have less proportionate costs, located in other parts of the country, but in no way is the service given comparable to the service in Glen Lake.[4]

Because of cost-cutting measures, a 1931 surplus of $8,033.16 carried over into the 1932 operating year. A financial crisis loomed, however, because only 11.83 percent of the patients were able to contribute toward their own care. The maximum charge allowed per week was twenty-one dollras, an increase of fourteen dollars since 1916, but the state aid contribution needed to cover costs for non-payers had not changed since then. It was still only five dollars per week. Even when supplemented by tax appropriations from Hennepin County, the public funding was inadequate to reimburse the weekly costs not covered by the patients who had no money. Thus, it was not good news that the 1932 budget was again being cut, this time by ten percent.[5]

Ever since the sanatorium's opening, the employees had enjoyed a number of perks, some of them justified on the basis of keeping them healthy and tuberculosis-free. In May of 1932, the employees lost their access to free medication, along with any laboratory or X-ray work, except for their annual exam.

While the sanatorium staff was coping with cuts, they learned that the 1933 budget would also be cut, by twelve percent.[6] The dietary department contributed mightily. It reduced food costs and waste to achieve a forty-percent decrease since the 1929 budget, achieving a cost of only fourteen cents per meal. Soups and salads were sent out on trays by request only. Patients were charged for extra portions of juices and ice cream.[7]

The laundry lessened its work load by ceasing to handle any clothing that required special handling, such as lace trim, crêpe de Chine, or any black or highly colored material. Some women in the West Cottage saw this as an entrepreneurial opportunity and earned money by hand-laundering fine lingerie and fabrics for other patients.[8]

Other savings were achieved because graduate nurses were willing to work for the pay of a practical nurse. Employees at the sanatorium considered themselves fortunate to have a job during the Depression. Mary Coover didn't want to work at a tuberculosis sanatorium, but her mother told her she had to take the job. The family had two more kids to educate, and there were no other chances for employment. Mary stayed for thirty-five years.[9]

While the sanatorium was able to lower per diem costs to $2.42 in 1932 and $2.24 in 1933, those savings were offset by a lowered tax appropriation from Hennepin County. The sanatorium closed the 1932 books with a surplus of seventy-four cents. The next year ended with the first ever deficit—$10,202.98.

Cost-saving measures continued. The pharmacists manufactured more and more of the preparations used at the sanatorium, saving $459 on cough mixtures alone. Charging employees for medications brought in $1,600. In the X-ray department, a home-built fluoroscope replaced one that broke. Because spending was limited to necessities, a clever seamstress fashioned faux velvet curtains for the auditorium stage by sewing together worn blankets and dying them a dark wine color.[10]

The seamstress wasn't the only one making do with materials on hand. Dr. Petter worked with maintenance employee Alan Dean to adapt existing tools and equipment. By grinding down the pinchers of pliers they created "handy bone-grasping forceps." Dean also cut down the sacral rest of a Hawley table to accommodate smaller-sized children, and he adapted a spinal frame called a Goldthwaite iron by bending it to facilitate the application of body casts for children. These efforts saved money while making children as comfortable as possible during necessary procedures.[11]

In some departments, the austerity measures caused workloads to increase. Social services thoroughly investigated residency and financial qualifications to make sure that patients who could pay would do so. Staff described the process as disheartening and practically useless because many of the applicants were already homeless or dependent on relief agencies for support.

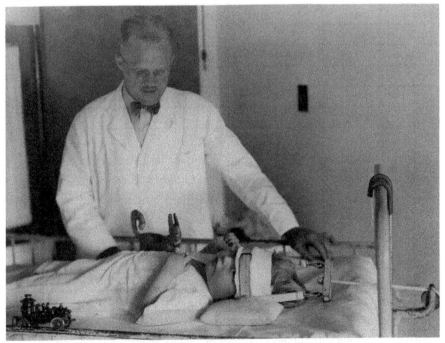

Dr. Petter with child. (Courtesy of the Hennepin History Museum)

The bad news from the economy was tempered by some good news, however. Medical experts had long claimed that one of the greatest benefits of a sanatorium was the removal of the open, infectious case from the community. Tables in Glen Lake's 1932 to 1933 report laid out numbers that supported the contention.[12]

Category	1916	1933
Death rate in Minnesota per 100,000	106	38
Death rate in Minneapolis per 100,000	147	37
New TB cases reported to Minneapolis Health Department	1,147	700

The number of new cases of tuberculosis in all forms reported in Minneapolis during 1933 was a significant drop from that of 1916, in spite of an increase in population. Dr. Mariette provided a table to demonstrate his belief that increasing the number of beds in a sanatorium facility correlated to a decline in the death rate.[13]

Ratio of Glen Lake Sanatorium beds to tuberculosis deaths in Minneapolis

Year	Beds	Total Deaths	Rate	Ratio of beds to death
1916	230	521	147	0.44
1925	620	348	81	1.8
1927	760	337	76	2.25
1932	760	207	43	3.6
1933	760	183	37	4.6

In the same report, he noted that Glen Lake had almost halved the death rate of its own patients. This improvement happened even though the sanatorium's mission was to treat far-advanced and moderately advanced cases of TB. Mariette attributed the gains to changes in surgical treatment and a better understanding of rest and diet.[14]

Category	1925*	1933
Percentage of patients discharged by death	38%	19%
Percentage of discharged arrested or apparently arrested	46%	74%
Percentage leaving without improvement or against advice	16%	7%

*1925 is when the main building and wings became fully operational

The sanatorium's reputation for success in tuberculosis treatment and patient care grew. In 1930, the Medical Research Committee of the National Tuberculosis Association selected Glen Lake as one of their research institutions. It was one of eighteen units in the United States chosen for this work. In addition to national research, individual physicians at the sanatorium conducted studies to determine the best treatments for tuberculosis. Topics ranged from TB of the ear to tuberculous laryngitis to cardiac lesions. In 1931, staff published twelve papers in medical journals and gave thirty-two presentations to local and regional organizations.

Supporting all of this research was the Medical Records Department. By 1931, the department had complied with the American College of Surgeon's minimum requirements for medical records. In 1934, the medical records personnel qualified as registered medical record librarians—among the first in the state. In 1937, the Standard Classified Nomenclature of Disease took the place of Glen Lake's version. The medical library and statistical department were then brought together into one office that analyzed statistics and prepared reports for the various government offices and tuberculosis organizations. The department consisted of two salaried employees and two patients working part time as preparation for discharge, an unusual staffing complement for a tuberculosis sanatorium.

Personnel from other sanatoriums came to Glen Lake for instruction and inspiration. In 1930, two Sisters of Charity (Gray Nuns) from St. Boniface Sanatorium near Winnipeg spent much of the year touring sanatoriums in the United States. They were in Minnesota for three months and chose Glen Lake as a model for their hospital, built in 1931.[15]

A well-known tuberculosis specialist is supposed to have called Glen Lake the "Mayo of Tuberculosis."[16] A collaborative relationship did exist between the sanatorium and the famous clinic in Rochester. Dr. H. Corwin Hinshaw, pulmonologist at Mayo, was an occasional consultant at the medical staff meetings. He helped establish an exchange fellowship that brought a different doctor to Glen Lake each month to spend a rotation studying the care of the tuberculous patients. Dr. Hinshaw was one of the first fellows. These fellowships expanded to bring physicians to Glen Lake from other continents, including Asia and South America, as well as from Canada and several states.

Along with the fiscal crises and professional successes, the staff faced an alcohol problem that grew worse after the Depression. When national pro-

Jack's Place ad. (Author's collection)

Kraemer's ad. (Author's collection)

hibition finally ended in 1933, local bars opened or reopened. Two establishments in the Glen Lake neighborhood on Excelsior Boulevard were within walking distance for up-patients. According to its ads, Jack's Place served the "Best Sandwiches in Glen Lake" and had Schmidt's, Gluek's, and Jordan on tap. Kraemer's was described as "rural Hennepin County's most popular café" and advertised Schmidt's and Miller's High Life beers.[17] Although hard liquor, such as whiskey or gin, was banned from the sanatorium, the possession of beer was merely "discouraged." Some visitors smuggled in a bottle or two for friends.

Many patients who had graduated to the cottages had friends with cars. For them, a favorite destination for a refreshing beverage was Pauley's Bar in Chanhassen.[18] Pauley's had pinball machines and also the advantage of being six miles away from the sanatorium and farther from the watchful eyes of neighbors than the establishments within walking distance. Glen Lake, which had been built far away from residential neighborhoods, was slowly being surrounded by housing. People who chose to build near a tuberculosis institution were now complaining about its function and its patients.

During the Depression, the consumption of liquor became closely associated with a lifestyle characterized by poor diets and equally poor living conditions. In late 1932, the Union Gospel Mission in Minneapolis reported that it was serving 1,800 homeless men daily. The Gateway District, a convergence of Hennepin, Nicollet, and Washington avenues, had become a haven for transients and the jobless.[19] Many of them turned to liquor for solace. The Gateway was also a breeding ground for tuberculosis. A tuberculous derelict brought to Minneapolis General Hospital would be sent out to Glen Lake. Some also arrived from the Salvation Army or the Federal Transient Camp at Savage, Minnesota.[20]

After being at the sanatorium for a while, the need for alcohol caused some patients to go absent without leave and head back to the Gateway. Many were eventually returned to the sanatorium, sometimes under the influence. A few became extremely boisterous and too much for the nursing staff to handle, prompting a call to the sheriff. Local law enforcement officers were reluctant to jail people with tuberculosis, however, and often released them, contributing to the cycle.

The sanatorium was still acting under the tuberculosis control law of 1913, which gave health officers the power to send to the sanatorium those people whom they judged to be health menaces. These incidents were commonly referred to as commitments, although they were seldom a court-ordered commitment as in the case of the state's mental hospitals. In a five-year period during the 1930s, there were fifty-eight commitment admissions to Glen Lake. That included eight repeat offenders who deserted and were committed a second or third time.

Desertion was relatively simple, with transportation from the sanatorium being the major hurdle. If they felt well enough to walk, they could merely choose a time to unobtrusively slip away from the building. A few asked for permission to leave. If they did, were denied, and left anyway, their discharge was noted as being "against medical advice" instead of desertion. The three-time deserter asked again for permission to leave, and his discharge was noted as "acquiesced." The doctors may have just given up.

Nine of the patients committed during that time period in the 1930s died. Sixteen stayed long enough to render their tuberculosis inactive and be recommended for discharge. Some were found to not be residents of Hennepin County and were transferred to other sanatoriums. Four others misbehaved so badly that they received a disciplinary discharge, with one of them going to jail.[21]

Because most of the disciplinary problems were caused by men living on One East, administration decided to convert room 186 East into a detention area. Windows were barred, and a double door installed. The inner "gate door" had an opening at the bottom where food on trays could be slipped to the "inmate." The room contained a toilet stool, a wash basin, and bunk beds. Staff commonly referred to this drying-out place as the jail or the drunk tank.[22]

Nurse Phyllis Burns remembered the time a patient who was a former professional boxer became drunk and wanted to fight everybody. He was put in the jail, and when the evening supervisor went to let him out, she found he had turned on the water and flooded the floor. She shut the door again, and the patient created such a disturbance that she finally called one of the doctors to help her. He looked at the situation and said, "Oh, that's just a boyish prank." When he went to open the door, the drunk patient said, "And just who are you, you bald-headed son-of-a-bitch?" Then it was a different story, she recalled—no longer just a boyish prank.[23]

Rules for the companion addiction, smoking, also tightened because too many patients were still smoking in bed. Smoking in general increased rather than decreased. Medical staff members were especially concerned that social service staff members routinely distributed Bull Durham tobacco and cigarette papers. They requested that the department stop this practice. Eventually, the sanatorium designated specific smoking rooms, and the physicians were advised to further set an example for the patients by not smoking while on duty.[24]

Pregnancy was another continuing concern. Glen Lake was part of the twenty-one percent of U.S. sanatoriums equipped to care for women throughout their pregnancy and labor.

From July 1934 to December 1939, twelve babies were born at the sanatorium, two of them to unmarried mothers. To try to settle the discussion of whether pregnancy could harm a tuberculous woman, the sanatorium researched 470 female patients who had been at Glen Lake over an eight-year period. Those who had borne children were compared to those who were never pregnant. The study, completed in 1937, showed very slight differences in health status, and the doctors concluded that pregnancy did not have a marked effect on the progress of tuberculosis.[25]

As a precaution, though, the sanatorium began to offer birth control information to all married women going home on leaves of absence. Those wanting to know more were referred to Dr. Lovett or Dr. Hutchinson, two female physicians on staff. This was a fairly radical move in the 1930s. Public health campaigns, along with the birth control movement headed by Margaret Sanger, had encouraged some changes in attitude, but the American Medical Association didn't incorporate contraception into medical school curriculum until 1937. The physicians at Glen Lake considered birth control to be a legitimate component of maintaining good health in a woman recovering from tuberculosis and acted accordingly.[26]

Although medical personnel came from around the world to study at Glen Lake, the University of Minnesota's tuberculosis instruction for medical students was curtailed. Harold S. Diehl, dean of the University of Minnesota medical sciences, become concerned about the rate of tuberculosis infections in fourth-year medical students. In 1937, a study revealed that among the university's medical school classes from 1919 to 1932, ninety-two students, or seven percent, developed clinical tuberculosis while in school or soon after graduation, and eleven died. As a result, the compulsory sanatorium teaching service at Glen Lake was discontinued and presented as an option.[27]

The university findings were disputed by a 1938 article written by Dr. Jennings of Glen Lake. His study found that none of the 526 students who had been at Glen Lake for the period of study had died of tuberculosis.[28] His unstated implication is that the students' active infection occurred during service at other university affiliates. Regardless of study results, by 1939, no medical students chose a sanatorium experience as a training option.[29] In succeeding years, some students were at the sanatorium as interns, but never again at the previous levels of participation.

This loss may have been a mixed blessing for Glen Lake. The medical staff meeting minutes contain remarks about the challenges of keeping the live-in interns on track for their term. Interns were sometimes absent on Sunday mornings and all of them were frequently out in the evening. One staff doctor commented that interns should be given more work to do so that they would have less time to play pool.[30]

With so many changes and adversities occurring at Glen Lake, patient dissatisfaction was growing. It was good that more people were leaving healed, but the Great Depression had caused high unemployment rates. People were eager to resume normal life and, for husbands and fathers of the 1930s, that included supporting their families. Dr. Mariette and his staff were concerned about men who would return to previous jobs of physical labor, experience a breakdown, and return to Glen Lake. Many of the patients were simply unable to return to their previous occupations.

In addition, it was difficult for ex-sanatorium patients to find new jobs when employers could choose from applicants without a work gap on their résumé. When that work gap was suspected to be related to tuberculosis, ex-patients were often not hired.

For some patients, the discrimination started even before discharge. If a patient was granted a leave longer than thirty-six hours and planned to stay in a private home, a notice was sent to the Department of Health, and a representative could choose to visit the home to ensure that necessary steps were taken to prevent contagion. In some cases, the patient would give up leave rather than embarrass his friends by having a visit from a health nurse.[31]

In 1937, a patient who was leaving against advice planned to rent an apartment. In accordance with laws regarding leaving against advice, the sanatorium informed the Department of Health, so it could inform the landlord of requirements to clean the apartment according to its regulations when the renter left. Some landlords changed their minds about the avail-ability of rooms when informed of the requirement.[32]

A newly discharged patient, then, could face two hurdles: where to live and how to earn a living. The social work, therapy, and education depart-ments at Glen Lake developed some solutions internally and also worked with various state and public agencies to provide solutions.

During their stay at Glen Lake, some patients had contributed what they could to their family by earning "pin money" through the sale of articles made in occupational therapy. Others chose to work at the sanatorium for pay as part of their discharge plan. Both of these options continued to be debated in medical journals. In any case, the earnings from either were rarely significant enough to replace a salary that could support a family.

The vocational and outpatient departments were primarily responsible for solving the employment dilemmas. In so doing, they worked with state organizations and learned from the experiences of similar institutions. The system they developed became a model for other sanatoriums.

14

Progress in the 1930s

ATTEMPTS TO FIND EMPLOYMENT PLACEMENTS for discharged patients were stymied by the lack of suitable situations for someone who needed to ease back into a normal work week. Those who had previously worked around dust, perhaps in one of the flour mills in Minneapolis, needed to find a less hazardous job. People who tested positive for TB couldn't work around food in a grocery store or restaurant. Even though a doctor affirmed that a meat handler with inactive TB was not a public health menace, the ex-patient could not return to his occupation without special permission from the Department of Health.[1]

Employees working in the sanatorium's programs of education and vocational training did their best to prepare patients for different occupations. It was especially challenging to help those patients with minimal education who could no longer perform a laborer's job. Formal education for many people, especially women, ended at the completion of eighth grade. It is estimated that only twenty percent of the U.S. population had a high school diploma at that time.[2]

The Division of Vocational Rehabilitation of the State Department of Education had provided a rehabilitation counselor to state and county sanatoriums starting in 1919, but educational services to patients were limited to correspondence courses.[3] Completion of those depended on the patient's perseverance. In 1929, the Minneapolis Public School Adult Education program was inaugurated at Glen Lake under the directorship of Katherine M. Kohler, with 200 patients enrolled. The Hennepin County Tuberculosis Association assisted by organizing a Glen Lake Education Committee and contributing to the salary of a full-time librarian.[4,5]

In order to accommodate these activities, spaces for education were included in plans for the sanatorium's last facility expansion. The top floor of the 1931 vocational annex housed a laboratory and four modern surgical suites, but the other floors contained an expanded occupational therapy department and several classrooms. The sanatorium was able to offer vocational classes in tailoring, cobbling, printing and barbering. Schoolrooms had typewriters and other business machines that provided hands-on experience with office equipment.[6]

Full credit toward a high school diploma was given for public school courses completed. There were no registration fees and books were furnished, but everyone needed a physician's permission to register for a class. The teacher came to the room of a patient who was on strict bed rest. Patients with wheelchairs attended class in the Vocational Building. As many as four full-time teachers taught at the sanatorium, assisted by qualified patients who were well enough to teach part time.

Clarence Bowers was the first to graduate from the educational program in 1934. He had been a freshman at Edison High School when diagnosed with tuberculosis. After a short time at the state sanatorium at Ah-gwah-ching, Clarence transferred to Glen Lake, where he was able to take credits in German, history, English, civics, and elementary science.[7]

Commencement exercises were held in the auditorium. For young people whose high school education was interrupted, the educational program's diploma could be from their home school. Pupils from the Children's Building and some adult patients received eighth-grade certificates at the ceremony. The staff and students celebrated Graduation Day with a dinner and speeches in the dining room.[8]

Naturalization classes were added to help immigrants become American citizens. Lip-reading instruction was included for the hard of hearing and for patients who had TB of the throat or ear.[9] A special home economics department was set up to aid young married women because the National Tuberculosis Association identified this group as being most likely to relapse. Regular classes covered different phases of homemaking, such as nutrition, food preparation, meal planning, household equipment, and clothing construction. The class was intended to help homemakers perform tasks more efficiently and with the least expenditure of time, money, and energy. Men were permitted to take the class, but few did.[10]

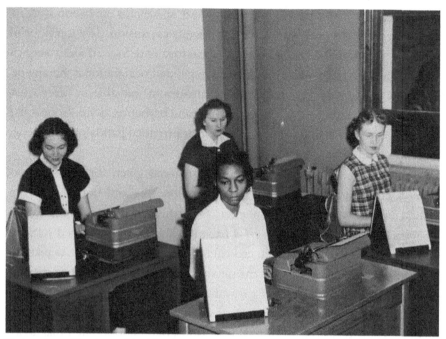

Typing class. (Courtesy of the Minnesota Historical Society)

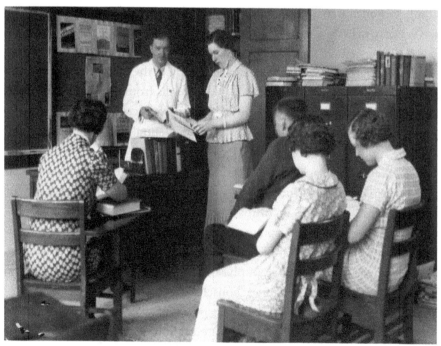

Teaching. (Courtesy of the Hennepin History Museum)

The testing bureau of the Minneapolis Adult Education Department administered psychological and intelligence quotient tests to help determine aptitudes and appropriate coursework. In 1932, a patient who had been a laborer at an ice dock was found to have a very high IQ and high clerical and vocabulary ratings. His training was tailored to his abilities, and he was hired as a record investigator for a mortgage company after discharge.[11]

In addition to the formal studies, public forums were broadcast over the radio system so strict bed patients could participate in learning. Topics were presented by university professors, a chief justice of the Minnesota Supreme Court, journalists from local newspapers, and physicians.

The patients in the printing and bookbinding classes on the ground floor of the new annex printed almost all of the sanatorium's forms and stationery: 40,000 nurses' reports each year; 20,000 envelopes; 50,000 laundry slips; 12,000 laboratory forms; and 60,000 medicine cards. They cut all of the typewriting paper to size, too.[12]

The vocational training class became an important part of the sanatorium's social life, as well. In 1933, the idea of a monthly in-house magazine was resurrected by the Trudeau Club, which wanted to produce a commemorative paper for the homecoming event. A contest to name the paper was announced over KNUT. The winning title, *Terrace Topics*, played off the name of the post office, Oak Terrace. The first issue was designed and printed at Glen Lake and given free to patients and visitors on August 26 at the first homecoming.

Terrace Topics met an important need and flourished. In less than a year, it went from a newspaper-style newsletter to a professionally printed magazine of 800 subscribed copies. The size of the magazine varied, with the smallest issue at sixteen pages and the largest at sixty. The task of printing that many copies became overwhelming, however, and later issues were produced by a print shop in Hopkins. Linoleum-block-print covers were designed by patients and printed at the sanatorium, sometimes in multiple colors. The covers and pages were then assembled and stapled by patients.[13]

The content was almost equally divided among informative articles, gossip columns, and original poems and short stories. Medical staff took turns contributing original articles, and there was an ongoing question-and-answer column, usually written by doctors Mariette or Mattill. Each issue listed the admissions and discharges for the previous month.

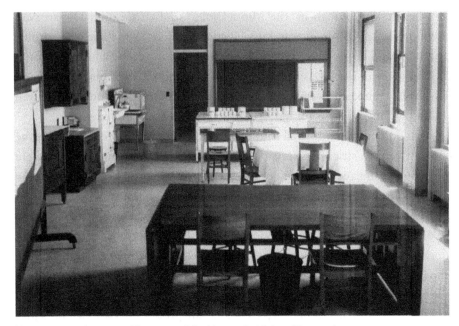

Home economics room. (Courtesy of the Hennepin History Museum)

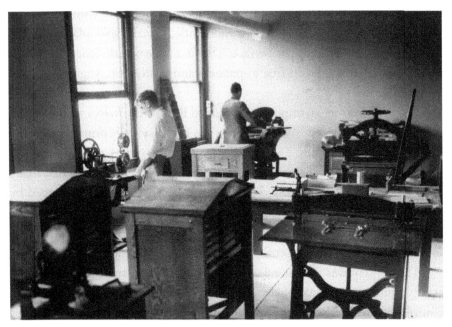

The print shop. (Courtesy of the Minnesota Historical Society)

Patients constituted the entire staff. The top post of editor went to an up-patient and changed almost monthly because he or she would be discharged from the sanatorium. Costs were covered with paid advertising from local businesses and yearly subscriptions. Bed patients sold subscriptions and ads by telephone. The annual subscription rate by mail was seventy-five cents; in-house was fifty cents. Single-copy issues cost five cents. Some patients earned business experience by doing the magazine's bookkeeping.

In order to give everyone a chance at working on *Terrace Topics*, the reporting staff changed each month, too. Patients gathered news and gossip from the ten wards. The gossip columns carried headings like "Back Fence Chatter," "San Jottings," and "Dishing out the Dirt." In "Keeping up with the Carrolls," the February 1936 issue said that Dr. William Carroll had a new Ford, Esther Carroll had a new permanent hair-do, and Russell Carroll had a new heartthrob. The heartthrob was Betty Wilke, who started employment at Glen Lake that year as one of two social workers serving 700 patients. She married Russell in November.[14]

The Children's Building had its own reporters, too. The older children were encouraged to write about school field trips and games in the "Kiddies Review" page. Gloria Stromseth Maxson was a patient in the Children's Building for thirteen years, until 1937. During that time she was a frequent contributor to *Terrace Topics*. Post-sanatorium, she became a teacher and published a book of poetry in 1974. One of her poems, titled "Nutritionist," may have been influenced by the Glen Lake dieticians.[15]

Terrace Topics also solicited original stories and poems from adult patients. The August 1935 issued contained Don Rivers's short story, "A Gentleman in Bed: The Episode of the Lady in Blue." Written in the style of Dorothy Sayers's stories of Lord Peter Wimsey, it relates the tale of a young man who instructs his manservant to communicate via flashlight and mirror with a young woman in a frothy blue nightgown who lives across the courtyard.[16] Rivers later had a career in marketing, working for the Knox-Reeves Advertising Agency as a copywriter.[17]

Working for the magazine gave many patients practical experience they could put on a résumé, but a source of immediate employment was created for some patients who seemed unemployable. The Hennepin County Sanatorium Commission members noticed that routine tasks at the sanatorium were being performed by personnel overpaid for that level of work. The

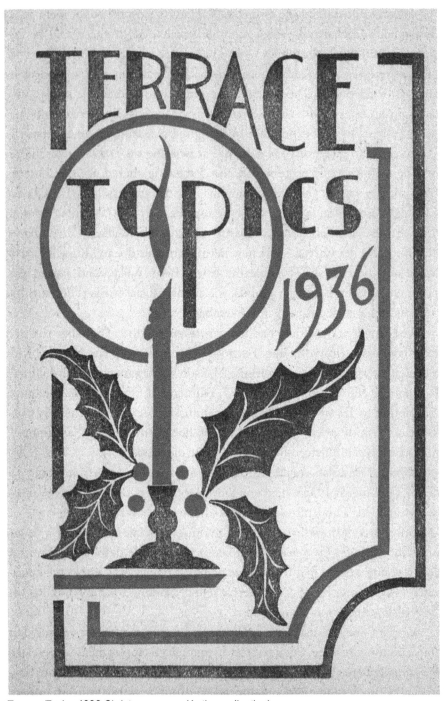

Terrace Topics 1936 Christmas cover. (Author collection)

commissioners decided to offer those jobs to ex-patients who could work four or more hours a day. They received room and board in the Employees' Building and earned a small salary of five or ten dollars per month.

The jobs consisted of light work and varied considerably. Ex-patients framed pictures in occupational therapy, tracked maintenance work requests, distributed library books, operated the elevators, and prepared specimen slides for lectures.

Dr. Mariette reported that it worked well, with an added bonus: "It has given suitable individuals a chance to 'harden up' under close medical supervision and so has enabled us to discharge a few patients earlier than we could otherwise."[18]

Most patients used the temporary jobs as a bridge to independence, but some patients never sought employment elsewhere once they had begun working at the sanatorium. For those whose family ties had been unraveled by tuberculosis, the relationships established during a multi-year stay were an acceptable substitute. One patient who became a long-term employee called it a second home.[19] For others, it may have been the familiarity of surroundings and the relief of not having to hide their tuberculous past.

Evelyn Romatko, who was shunned at a family reunion, remained at the sanatorium as an employee for more than twenty years. As a bed patient, she earned her high school diploma. When she became an up-patient, she worked in the sanatorium store, scooping ice cream and selling items to fellow patients. She also worked at the telephone switchboard as an ex-patient before being hired by the occupational therapy department and working there until her retirement.[20]

Jim Dragotis was a patient for two and a half years and married a nurse, Margaret, who had worked in both the children's and main buildings. He was hired to work in the storeroom. When asked how it felt to start working after being on the cure, he said, "I felt like a million dollars." [21]

For women, the stigma of TB meant that nursing often became the best career for them.[22] Some already intended to be nurses but when they came to the sanatorium as student nurses, they contracted TB and became patients themselves.[23] Arlene Geuder was one of them. She finished nurse's training after her discharge. She returned to Glen Lake as a nurse, met her future husband at the sanatorium, and worked there a total of twenty years.[24]

Ruth Soland Altland was exposed to tuberculosis via her maternal grandmother, who stayed six months in each of her six children's homes. The widow's "asthma" turned out to be tuberculosis, and as many as ten grandchildren may have died from TB. Ruth was attending Minneapolis Business School when an X-ray showed shadows on her lung. Ruth was sure she would die from TB, too. Fortunately, she was counseled by a head nurse in her ward who had been a patient and willingly showed her scars and talked about the surgery. As an up-patient, she typed the manuscript for Dr. Wilmer's book, *Huber the Tuber*. Ruth was discharged in 1940, determined to be a nurse. She entered Hamline University's nursing program on a scholarship and earned a degree. She worked at Glen Lake for a short time before moving out of state.[25]

Not all women became nurses. Pernilla Lembke, who entered Glen Lake in 1933 and attended high school classes while a patient, went on to graduate with distinction from the University of Minnesota with a Bachelor of Science degree. She later obtained a Master's of Social Work from the University of Pennsylvania.[26]

Olga Saari chose employment at the sanatorium. Before becoming a patient, she graduated from Paul's Beauty School and worked in a Minneapolis salon. She established a beauty shop at the sanatorium and accommodated her clients, whether they were in wheelchairs, litters, or beds. She was a living example of her motto, "To look well is to feel well."[27]

Margaret Rutherford also chose to work at Glen Lake. She entered as a patient in 1921, and in 1962 she looked back at her bout with tuberculosis as a "lucky" break. "Working at Glen Lake was my compensation," she told a reporter. She spent thirty-seven and a half years at the sanatorium as the administrative secretary to three successive Glen Lake administrators. Rutherford said she held back tears when she arrived as a patient and again when she left as a retiree.[28]

Alfred Greene, the wizard with the radio system, spent almost three years at Glen Lake as a patient. He finished his education after discharge, but his goals had changed. Instead of becoming an engineer, he returned to the sanatorium as an X-ray technician and instructor. Green served at various times as the president, executive secretary, and treasurer of the American Society of Radiographers. He also edited *The X-Ray Technician*, a national magazine. When he resigned from Glen Lake, his position was filled by Ray McInnis, another former patient.[29]

A different employment/housing option was offered to ex-patients who wanted to work outside the sanatorium setting. In 1927, the Hennepin County Tuberculosis Association had established a boarding club at 1520 Park Avenue in the former home of Judge Martin B. Koon. The sixteen-room mansion was meant to solve temporary housing problems by giving free home care. The fourteen discharged patients who lived there were expected to leave once they found a job and a place to live.

In 1930, the association was deeded 1827 Portland Avenue by Francisca (Mrs. W.O.) Winston. The boarding club moved there, and the home was named Sarahurst in honor of the donor's mother and daughter. Local organizations sponsored remodeling and provided furnishings. The house, maintained by Christmas seals proceeds, could provide room and board for about fifteen ex-patients. The mission changed slightly, with most of the residents acquiring post-secondary education or being trained for jobs at Dunwoody Institute and other schools.[30]

In 1943, a study of forty-seven former residents of Sarahurst five years after discharge from the sanatorium found that forty-three were well and working. Four ex-patients had returned to Glen Lake for further treatment, but none had died. This compared to a national average of twenty percent

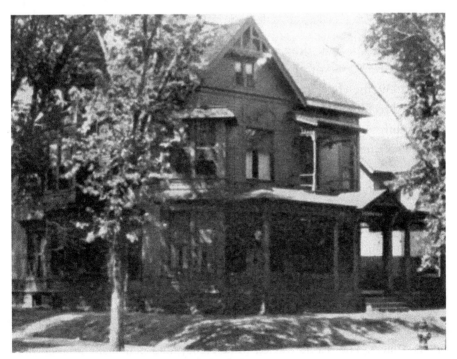

Boarding Club. (Courtesy of the Lokke Collection)

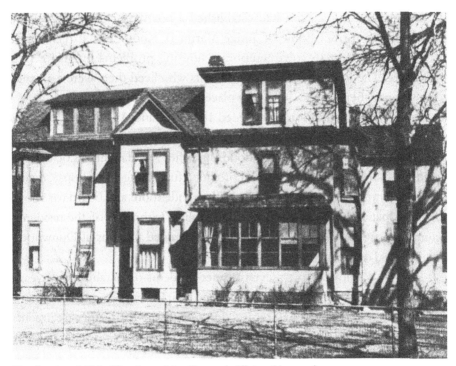

The Sarahurst Club. (Courtesy of the Hennepin History Museum)

of former TB patients dead after five years. The study emphasized the importance of a period of aftercare between discharge and self-support.

In 1939, the Hennepin County Tuberculosis Association of Minneapolis turned to filmmaking to publicize its success in vocational rehabilitation. Sanatorium scenes for the color motion picture *Restored* were filmed at Glen Lake. The fifteen-minute movie followed a factory girl from development of tuberculosis through sanatorium treatment, education within the sanatorium, retraining at Sarahurst, home care, and return to self-support. The film debuted at the Southern Tuberculosis Conference in Charleston, South Carolina.[31] In September of that year, Rosetta van Gelder from the department of rehabilitation of the National Tuberculosis Association visited Sarahurst and Glen Lake. She commented that in no other city had she found a plan equal in effectiveness to the one worked out in Minneapolis and Glen Lake.[32]

Life wasn't all work and no play, though. Other things were happening at Glen Lake, including annual visits by baseball players from the Minneapolis Millers. The team's owner, Mike Kelley, had personally granted permission for the games to be rebroadcast to the bed patients when the live game was during rest hours. In 1935, Joe Hauser and Andy Cohen from the Minneapolis Millers visited the children's camp and the children's building. Both players promised to hit homes runs at that afternoon's game, and both did. Halsey Hall, the baseball announcer for WCCO, mentioned that in his broadcast of the game.[33] Ted Williams visited in 1938, the year he played for the Millers before being called up to the big leagues.

Irving Sandler, who entered the sanatorium in 1936, described himself as having connections in show business. Other accounts say that he had in fact been a successful tap dancer on the vaudeville circuit. Although Sandler was

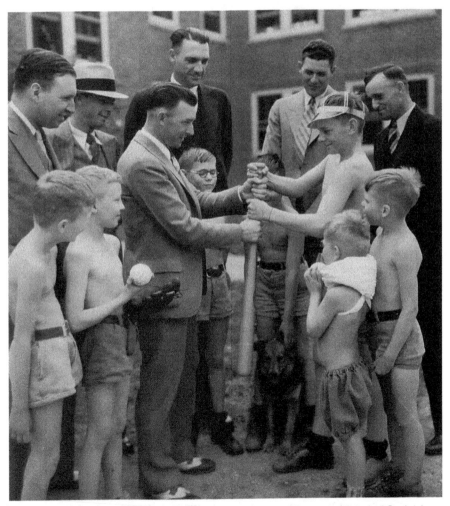

The Minneapolis Millers with Ted Williams. (Courtesy of the Minnesota Historical Society)

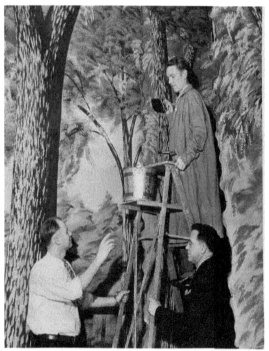

on strict bed rest for more than two years, he used some of his connections to persuade entertainers to come out to Glen Lake for shows.[34] The Variety Club of the Twin Cities, a social organization of men in show business, also brought programs to the sanatorium. That included a local premier of the film *Rhodes of Africa*, about Cecil Rhodes and South Africa, in the summer of 1936.[35]

Mrs. George C. Christian brought a different type of entertainment to Glen Lake when she sponsored presentations of classical music. In 1935, many patients crowded into the auditorium to hear the

Waldo and the auditorium backdrop. (Courtesy of the Minnesota Historical Society)

Minneapolis Symphony Orchestra under the direction of Eugene Ormandy.[36] In 1938, it was the Twin Cities Philharmonic Society that she arranged to give a performance at the sanatorium.[37]

There were improvements to the sanatorium campus in the 1930s, some of them due to the Federal Works Progress Administration program. The auditorium gained an impressive backdrop thanks to Helmer Gunnarson, a patient-artist who did the medical drawing for Glen Lake. His former art instructor, Charles S. Wells, directed the Minneapolis Art Project. He hired Stanley Waldo to design and paint a screen, and it served as a stage background for six decades.[38]

Following tradition, performers would sign the backs of scenery boards. One of the scrawled signatures on the old backdrop was of Bill "Bojangles" Robinson, probably written in the 1920s when he was part of the Orpheum circuit.[39]

In 1936, several Glen Lake workers voted to unionize, a move that would alter the working relationship between them and administration. The union movement for public employees began in Wisconsin, after the National Industrial Recovery Act in 1933 and the National Labor Relations Act in 1935 provided for collective bargaining. In 1936, the American Federation of Labor officially recognized the American Federation of State, County, and Municipal Employees. Secretaries, maintenance people, and dietary workers at Glen Lake joined fellow public hospital workers in this new union. With the effects of the Great Depression easing and other employment opportunities becoming available, the employees began to question workplace conditions. One result was Dr. Mariette's request to the sanatorium commission for approval of a forty-hour work week.[40]

In the absence of a cure for tuberculosis, physicians continued to develop surgical interventions to hasten a patients' recovery. On July 20, 1937, Dr. Thomas J. Kinsella was the first Minnesota physician to successfully remove a cancerous lung. In December, he removed a tuberculous lung. Lobectomies (removal of one or more lobes) and pneumonectomies (removal of an entire lung) were last-resort surgeries because the risk of infection was great and there were only sulfanilamides, no penicillin or other antibiotics. There was also the danger that the surgery could cause the tuberculosis to spread, and the patient would be sicker after surgery than before.[41]

Quack medicine had been a problem at Glen Lake since it opened. People suffering with consumption were the targets of advertisements for many questionable medications that offered to cure the disease. These unregulated syrups and pills could be ordered from catalogs, including that of Sears, Roebuck and Company. A tuberculous person could chose from products such as tar expectorant to strengthen the lungs or Curtis's Consumption Cure that would "control the organization of food material."[42]

Although the Food and Drugs Act of 1906 required labels to disclose dangerous ingredients, the Supreme Court ruled in 1911 that the act's wording did not prohibit false claims. This allowed for the continued sale of hundreds of fraudulent medications. The doctors at Glen Lake would confiscate these mail-order drugs when found. Some were not merely ineffective, but contained some of those dangerous ingredients that needed to be listed—alcohol, heroin, and cocaine among them. The 1938 Food, Drug, and Cosmetic Act finally prohibited the marketing of drugs with false therapeutic claims, and fewer unauthorized medicines arrived at Glen Lake.

Patients were isolated physically from world events during the late 1930s but were kept informed through newspapers and magazines. Many corresponded with pen pals from sanatoriums in Canada and Europe. Chow Yoke Keng, a Chinese girl taking the cure in Tjiandoer, Java, wrote directly to *Terrace Topics*, which published her letters.[43]

Patients were well aware of the uncertainty and unrest that others were experiencing. They joined the British in celebrating the coronation of King George VI after the shock of his brother's abdication. In July 1937, they heard the Japanese invaded China. And they heard that Mussolini and Hitler were both supplying support troops for the Nationalists in the Spanish Civil War. News reports of the air raids in Spain awakened the World War I memories of patient George Scherling. The normally upbeat *Terrace Topics* published the thoughtful "Portrait of a Pacifist." The article recounted Scherling's life as a Jew under German rule in Lithuania and the bombing of Telz by Zeppelins. It mirrored the concern felt by patients as the U.S. government struggled to maintain neutrality.[44]

In June of 1939, a literal wind of change occurred when a small tornado hit the buildings. It caused little damage, and, in fact, the patients regarded it as beneficial. The wind stripped the leaves off the trees between the main building's wings, permitting clear views between the men's and women's floors.[45]

And so ended the 1930s. It was a decade that had begun well and then presented challenges, but at Glen Lake it ended with renewed vigor and optimism.

15

The World War II Years

O N January 1, 1940, Maryanna Shorba opened her diary, a Christmas gift, and wrote: "Here it is; a nice new one. The last is full of laughter and tears. This finds me in the San and where will it find me five years from now only God knows."[1]

The relative calm of the late 1930s extended into 1940 at Glen Lake, and so did the fight against tuberculosis, with continued hopes for a cure. The National Tuberculosis Association adopted a new tactic for educating the public and released an animated cartoon about the disease. *Goodbye, Mr. Germ* was directed by Edgar Ulmer, a Hollywood director with a unique visual style. He combined photographs with drawings to tell the adventures of a germ named "Tee Bee." The germ swims around from lung to lung, raising a family, until it finally gets trapped in a sanatorium. The film urged people to be aware of lingering coughs and to get tuberculin tests.[2]

Because of the 1938 drug act, self-medication was less of an issue at the sanatorium until several patients sent for a medication called tubercle antigen. Patients were instructed by mail how to administer the serum themselves. Their willingness to expose themselves to the danger of unsterile injections demonstrates the desperation felt by those who used it. The supplier was able to circumvent the mail-order restriction for several years because the drug was based on the tuberculin agent used for testing. Eventually, a Glen Lake laboratory technician ordered the product and tested it on guinea pigs. All of the guinea pigs receiving the antigen lost weight and died before any from the control group did. That finding defended the staff's confiscation of the product.[3]

Lung surgery was still a risky attempt to halt the disease, and Myrtle Johnson was among the first Glen Lake patients to have one of her lungs removed. She went to St. Mary's Hospital to have the surgery done by Dr. Kinsella in October 1940. Doctors Funk and Larson from the sanatorium assisted at the operation. She was on strict bed rest until the next April, when she transferred to Ah-gwah-ching. Myrtle would live almost fifty more years with just one lung.[4]

Not everyone would undertake the risk. After several failed pneumo-therapies were performed on Theresa Ledermann, Dr. Kinesella conferred with her father. Although there were some successes, a female patient from Glen Lake had recently died after having the surgery. That influenced her father's decision not to have Theresa undergo a lobectomy. They did a thoracoplasty instead. Theresa, a young teenager, had to wear a thoracic jacket night and day for three months. The canvas vest went across her chest and over a shoulder, with seven sponges placed in pockets to help push in her ribs. It was not comfortable, and it left her with a deformed ribcage.[5]

New equipment at the sanatorium included an up-to-date X-ray machine. An article in *Terrace Topics* compared the control panel to a submarine dashboard. Wires were shockproof, and the radiation tubes were enclosed in a chamber. Best of all, the table tilted to allow Lipiodol, a contrast agent, to run into the far reaches of the lung. No longer did patients need to nearly stand on their heads to obtain results.[6]

News of Germany's invasions in Western Europe reached the sanatorium, but immediate effects were few. One of the first consequences, oddly enough, was the unavailability of Lipiodol for use with the new X-ray machine. The poppyseed oil used as a radio-opaque contrast agent was processed in France.[7]

The somber tone of world events continued to be reflected in *Terrace Topics*. Worthy Turner submitted a serious essay titled "A Democratic Quirk." Turner was a musician who traveled and sang with Henry Thompson and his Negro Orchestra, based in Texas. Turner eloquently described his feelings about being a black person at Glen Lake by first asking, "Does America believe in democracy?"

I am one of a small minority in this institution and I'd like to relate some of my experiences in this so-called democracy of ours. . . . Right here in this San I can feel the presence of indifference in almost every social undertaking I go through. There are only two more of my race (patients) that are up and around and as they are somewhat my seniors I don't run into them except during mealtimes. Of course, when I meet members of your group, most of them nod me a brief "hello" and try to maintain a civil atmosphere. Naturally, I have built up a philosophical attitude. I don't think many of you feel superior to any one of us and I don't feel inferior to any one of you. In fact, I think that most of you would have difficulty in explaining your feelings on the subject; you are the victims of a feeling which has been bred into you as a complex. Our question was: Does America believe in democracy? If we really believe in it and expect to preserve it for any of us, we must believe in it for all of us, not merely for the rich and not the poor, the well-learned and not the illiterate, or all races excluding the Negro.[8]

Wilton Lofstrand, editor of the next issue, responded to Turner's article by noting, "most doctors pay more attention to what is inside of a patient's skin and the attitude of his mind than to reflect on the pigmentation of his skin, unless he happens to be a dermatologist." In the September issue, Lofstrand penned "Racial Prejudice," which pondered the social evil that seemed to be so hard to eliminate.[9]

Terrace Topics experienced a period of excellence in writing and art at this period in time. A series of editors with advanced educational degrees and/or journalistic experience solicited and encouraged original articles rather than relying on clip sheets from the National Tuberculosis Association. Dr. Earl Opstad was editor when George Scherling's article appeared. Opstad stayed on at Glen Lake as a staff doctor after his own recovery and discharge.[10]

Editor Maryanna Shorba, who would finish a journalism degree post-sanatorium, published Turner's essay. She wasn't the editor, though, when her future husband wrote "The Black Cat Murder" for the November 1941 issue.[11] Shorba and Frederick Manfred first met when their litters were next to each other in the hallways of Glen Lake. A former sports reporter for the *Minneapolis Journal* and an aspiring novelist, Manfred was discouraged from writing in the sanatorium. The doctors thought patients should plan for different work post-sanatorium and told him to go into something softer than the newspaper business. Manfred disagreed with them and submitted several stories and poems to the magazine.

Manfred later fictionalized his experience at Glen Lake in his novel *Boy Almighty*. The main character, Eric Frey, is based on a mixture of himself and one of his roommates. His physician, Dr. Sumner Cohen, reviewed the manuscript for accuracy and was a model for the book's Dr. Abraham. Manfred later said the time available for reading and analyzing other authors greatly benefitted him as an author.[12]

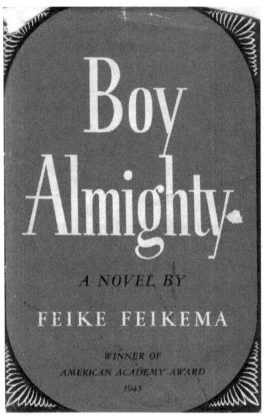

Manfred and his roommate Dr. Harry Wilmer created and wrote about anthropomorphic tuberculosis bacilli with similar names. Manfred (as Feike Feikema) published "Hubert the Tuber Complains," "Hubert the Tuber Discusses Human Dignity," and "Hubert the Tuber Encourages Revolt" in *Terrace Topics*.[13] Wilmer dropped the T from his germ's name, and *Huber the Tuber* was published by the National Tuberculosis Association in 1942. The Glen Lake medical staff endorsed it as being "clever as well as of excellent educational value to the average layman."[14] The NTA agreed, promoting the book to schools and children's hospitals. Huber, modeled after several bad guys of the era, including Hitler, was into a fourth printing by 1949.

Fred Manfred's *Boy Almighty* cover. (Author collection)

Writing was clearly an important outlet for many of the patients. Jean Mason, who researches health communication, discussed pathography (writing by patients) in her article "The Discourse of Disease." Mason studied writings produced by patients at Saranac Lake and examined how they used writing to document their experience, perhaps as a way to make sense of it.

"Within this environment [sanatorium], TB patients shared a common challenge—long hours of enforced idleness," she wrote. "A favorite way to fill this emptiness was to write."[15]

Maryanna Shorba continued to write in her diary nearly every day. Her sanatorium journey ended on July 8, 1941, when she wrote, "I am home!" She and Frederick Manfred married the next year.

On December 7, 1941, the plans and journeys of many people were put on hold. Almost every aspect of Glen Lake's operation experienced significant change when the bombing of Pearl Harbor brought the United States into World War II. The medical staff began granting special Christmas leave requests to patients whose relatives were drafted or had volunteered for service. One was from a patient who wasn't entitled to a leave, but her husband was home from the army for Christmas. Because the doctors agreed "she may never see him again," they granted a thirty-six-hour leave. As the war continued, special leaves were routinely approved.[16]

About forty employees resigned and joined the armed forces, but only two doctors on the medical staff were healthy enough to qualify for service. Dr. Victor Funk, a veteran of World War I, volunteered his services to the U.S. Navy Medical Corps. His commission in the U.S. Naval Reserve became effective in February 1942, and his first assignment was at the Mare Island Navy Hospital in California. The other enlistee was Dr. Golden Selin, who came to work at the sanatorium in 1941 and joined the Army Medical Corps in 1942.[17]

Not being able to serve in wartime was frustrating for men at the sanatorium who looked healthy but could not pass a physical for enlistment. Dr. Mariette told patients that the best way for them to serve their country consisted of staying well and not infecting

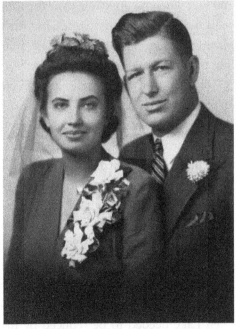

Fred and Maryanna Manfred. (University of Minnesota Anderson Library, Manfred archives))

others who could take a more active part in defense. Patients participated in the war effort by buying war saving stamps at the Oak Terrace Store. The stamps, available in ten-cent and twenty-five-cent versions, accumulated interest and could be redeemed for war bonds.[18]

The Office of Civilian Defense designated Glen Lake as a casualty receiving hospital, which included participating in black-outs and preparedness drills. The first simulated disaster drill on October 14, 1942, featured a Hopkins man with severe burns, a victim delivered in a grocery truck from Richfield, a maternity case, and four enemy aviators whose plane had been shot down near Mound.[19]

The airspace over Glen Lake was part of a flight path for pilots training for the Army Air Corps. When those men in their Piper Cubs discovered near-naked women sunbathing on the Four West porches, they started to buzz the sanatorium. They came down so low that Virginia Schwarting saw a plane from her room as the pilot pulled up sharply to clear the roof. Dr. Mariette called the Naval Air Station near Wold-Chamberlain Field, and they brushed off his complaint. One day a patient reported that a plane was down. Edward Thompson was flying at 150 miles per hour at a height of 500 feet when he dove low over the sanatorium and crashed into a tree. He walked away with slight injuries, but the plane burned. Thompson was disciplined for stunting with an airplane, but after that the planes were so far up that patients could hardly see them.[20]

Shortages of food and goods affected the sanatorium. One unexpected effect was the reduction of visiting hours. Because the Japanese controlled the rubber-producing areas of Asia, there was a shortage of rubber for tires. That in turn affected car owners and the bus lines, so fewer people visited.[21]

The dietary department cautioned staff and residents to be more careful with tableware, dishes, and glasses because merchandise would become more difficult to obtain and more expensive. Patients were asked to find some other way to salute new or graduate patients in the dining room rather than banging on tableware, because of the breakage of dishes.[22]

Rationing of such items as sugar, coffee, tea, cocoa, and spices began in the spring of 1942. As an institution, the sanatorium was permitted a use-percentage based on past orders. For instance, sugar consumption at Glen Lake needed to be reduced by fifty percent. The dietary department discontinued extremely sweet desserts and reduced sugar in others by using honey, syrup, or molasses intead. As *Terrace Topics* explained, "Sugar makes alcohol. Alcohol makes smokeless powder. Smokeless powder makes bullets. One pound of sugar will provide forty-seven bullets."[23]

It was relatively easy to accommodate the rationing of coffee, but change became imperative when meats, fats, and dairy products were added to the rationing list. Menus were simplified, with less variety and very few "special" meals. Townsend's rotating menu of seven differing entrées disappeared forever. She was not at Glen Lake to witness the dismantling of her innovations, having retired in November 1941. Other foods were not rationed, but were simply not available for a long time, including catsup.[24]

"Use it up, wear it out, make it do, or do without!" was the theme at most homes during the war. At Glen Lake, that meant cutting Sears Roebuck catalogs into squares to be used for sputum cups. Newspapers were folded into bedside waste bags.[25] Doctors experienced shortages when it was no longer possible to obtain the cellophane used in their surgical masks.[26]

The youngsters in the Children's Building did their part, too, by planting a victory garden to help with the food supply. Two up-patients partnered with a bed patient to plan and tend garden plots so all the children could participate.[27]

A Keep 'Em Happy Club supported the morale of former sanatorium employees in military duty. Each serviceman and servicewoman received the *Terrace Topics*, a subscription to *Reader's Digest*, a gift at Christmas, and correspondence from one of the club members. The club collected waste paper to raise funds for their treasury. The paper they sold varied in value, but for the first salvage drive the prices per hundred pounds were thirty-five cents for newspaper, seventy-five cents for cardboard, and forty-five cents for magazines. The club collected 1,500 pounds of paper in their first effort.[28]

The most serious shortage to affect the patients at Glen Lake was, by far, the lack of nursing personnel. Many nurses had volunteered for the Army or Navy nurse corps. Before the war started, the sanatorium's general duty nursing staff each day consisted of forty-two to fifty registered nurses, fifty-six practical nurses, and thirteen ward maids. In 1943, the nursing staff at Glen Lake cared for the same number of patients with only ten graduate or registered nurses, thirty-two practical nurses, four nursing aides, and thirteen ward maids.[29]

Some procedures not absolutely necessary to the welfare of the patients were discontinued. Intra-sanatorium visits to other patients via litter or wheelchair required someone to push them, so those were curtailed. Patients' beds were no longer rotated to provide equal opportunities for window views. Backrubs were given by physician order only. Non-health treatments, such as for dandruff, were discontinued. All daytime entertainments ceased for the duration of the war, except for Christmas and Easter celebrations.[30]

In 1942, Glen Lake chose to "home-grow" nurses and developed a course for nurses' aides, which included a stipend for attending. Five health attendants and twelve maids completed the course. Some took additional instruction and qualified as practical nurses. The courses were then offered to the general public. Of the total students completing the courses, eleven were still employed at the sanatorium a year later, at salaries of $100 per month.[31]

All hospitals were experiencing shortages, and the federal government was concerned about having a good supply of nurses near the battlefields. The United States Cadet Nurse Corps was created in 1943 to provide accelerated nursing training, during which the students would work in local hospitals. In exchange for the subsidized training, nurses were required to serve in areas of essential need at home or abroad for the duration of the war.

In Minneapolis, the first cadet nurse students were divided into groups and housed at various hospitals, including Minneapolis General, St. Mary's, the University of Minnesota, and Miller in St. Paul. Every three months they were rotated to another hospital to get specific training from each. They also had to spend two weeks at Glen Lake Sanatorium to learn about tuberculosis care.[32]

Several nurses came to Glen Lake permanently through that program. Beulah Baxter came as a cadet nurse and stayed until she retired. Phyllis Burns trained as a cadet nurse in Rochester, and then came to Glen Lake to fulfill her service obligation. She went back to Rochester to work, but returned to Glen Lake in 1947 and retired in 1966. Margaret Anderson went to nursing school in Minnesota and enrolled in the Cadet Nurse Corps for the last six months, which she spent at the Great Lakes Naval Hospital. From there she went to work at a veterans' hospital in Arizona, and then moved back with a friend to work at Glen Lake in the Children's Building until she, too, retired.[33]

The tuberculosis service for cadet nurses presented the same risks as the medical and nursing internships always had. Constance M. Otten, of Sioux City, Iowa, contracted tuberculosis during her training at either Minneapolis

General Hospital or Glen Lake Sanatorium. She was declared disabled in January 1947 because of the disease and filed a lawsuit for contracting tuberculosis during training. She sued the hospital and the Hennepin County Sanatorium Commission, but because she received a stipend of twenty dollars per month from the University of Minnesota, the state Supreme Court ruled that the university was responsible for compensation.[34]

Cadet nurses also came to Glen Lake from schools in other states, including the University of Missouri; the Sioux Valley Hospital in Sioux Falls, South Dakota; and the general hospital at Devils Lake, North Dakota.[35] Most of them worked on Five Administration, the "safe" floor, among the extra-pulmonary cases. In addition to the cadets, nursing students came to Glen Lake from Kahler Hospital School in Rochester, St. Barnabas in Minneapolis, St. Gabriel's in Little Falls, and Hibbing General. Charlotte Crowe did her field work at Glen Lake in 1945 while a student at the University of Manitoba. She worked in Saskatchewan for a while and was asked in 1949 if she wanted to return to Glen Lake as an assistant director of nurses. She did, and she would retire as director of nurses in 1977.[36]

The presence of cadet nurses and student nurses couldn't begin to alleviate the staff shortage at Glen Lake, and it wasn't just a nursing shortage, either. Other employees had left to work at defense industries for much higher salaries. Some former and retired employees, many of them elderly and unable to perform a full day's work, returned to work at the sanatorium as part of what they saw as a contribution to the war effort.[37]

A partial solution to the employee shortage came through negotiations with the War Relocation Authority, a U.S. government agency charged with relocating Japanese Americans to internment camps. Two nurses, two orderlies, and two waiters came to the sanatorium after having their background checked by the FBI, the Navy, and the war intelligence services. This was a controversial move. Glen Lake's union employees voted on a resolution to support the hiring and were evenly divided at twenty-three to twenty-three.[38]

Terrace Topics extended a hearty welcome to the Japanese nurses. "May you find your new homes and jobs at Glen Lake a relief from your confines," one issue read. "We'll do our best to see you won't be sorry you came to be with us and help us. We're certainly honored, we can tell you."[39]

Mona Takao was one of women who arrived in Minnesota from an internment camp. She enrolled in the nursing program at St. Joseph's Hospital in St. Paul and took further training at Minneapolis General Hospital, Fergus Falls State Hospital, and Glen Lake Sanatorium.[40]

Kimi Hara also arrived via the program. She was born in Seattle in 1915 and graduated from high school in 1933. She went to nursing school at Swedish Hospital in Seattle, graduated in 1940, and worked there for a time. After Pearl Harbor was bombed, she tried to join the Army Nurse Corps, but they wouldn't take her because she was Japanese. When the government started the internment camps, Japanese people east of the Rockies didn't have to go, so Kimi found a job at St. Mary's Hospital in Rochester in February of 1942. Her grandmother, aunt, and sister Reiko were then able to leave camp to join her in Rochester. Kimi developed tuberculosis and was admitted to Glen Lake as a patient. She continued her nursing career after discharge, and in 1956, Governor Orville Freeman appointed her to the State Board of Nursing.[41]

The first war-related refugee arrived at the sanatorium in November. Peter Mah, age nineteen, escaped from China via Hong Kong and arrived in Seattle. He was relocated to Minneapolis, but was found to have tuberculosis and was sent to Glen Lake.[42]

The war added to the workload at Glen Lake in many ways. Because the workforce shortages were universal, other county sanatoriums in Minnesota could no longer maintain their previous levels of surgical treatments. By 1942, only Nopeming and Glen Lake offered surgery. Patients came to Glen Lake from Fair Oaks Lodge, Buena Vista, Riverside, Deerwood, Otter Tail, and Sand Beach. The increase in surgeries and the workload of medical staff prompted Dr. Mariette to add patient care to his administrative duties, and he assumed responsibility for fifty-eight people.[43]

The war may have also resulted in a revised policy at Glen Lake for the distribution of patient information. Back in 1925, anyone could inquire about the status of a patient, in person or by telephone. Data privacy was not a common phrase or concept. Each patient had a card at the information booth in the reception area. Every morning, the cards were updated with the most recent information by the use of colored metal snaps attached to the cards indicating that a patient's condition was fair, good, poor, or serious. In 1933, a legal opinion had stated, "As the sanatorium is a public institution, its records are open to inspection by anyone desiring to make legitimate use of the information obtained."[44] The definition of "legitimate use" was open to interpretation and a patient's condition could be disclosed to almost anyone who called to ask.

An increased emphasis on secrecy ("Loose lips sink ships") may have inspired a new attitude toward information sharing. One of Glen Lake's legal sources cautioned the doctors to remember that the physician-patient relationship exists, and physicians were not allowed to give information to relatives. By 1942, Glen Lake was using a new form titled "Information Authorization." Patients were to approve access to their records by indicating "yes" or "no" to categories of people or institutions who might want access.[45]

Other issues arose. The educational system was nearly lost in 1942, when the attorney general ruled that the Minneapolis Board of Education could not pay salaries to teachers outside of their district. The board then withdrew its financial support. Later, the attorney general reversed that finding because the patients were living outside the school district for reasons beyond their control. The board resumed support by paying on a per-student tuition basis instead, and nine students graduated that year.[46]

While coping with shortages, Glen Lake was drawn into a local controversy that involved two serious illnesses—rheumatic fever and polio.

By the 1940s, doctors were aware that acute rheumatic fever could develop after a throat infection. In about half of those cases, long-term damage could occur to heart valves. Tuberculosis and rheumatic fever had a shared history in Minneapolis. In 1922, the Lymanhurst School for Tuberculosis had created a space for the care of children with rheumatic fever. The director, Dr. Morse Shapiro, was involved in research and therapy programs for the disease and received philanthropic support for his efforts. The Lymanhurst space was called the Variety Heart Clinic, in recognition of donations from the entertainment industry group.

Localized polio epidemics had appeared in the United States every summer since about 1916, when there were more than 2,000 deaths in New York City. Several therapies had been tried, but most of the effort went into developing devices to help survivors of polio cope with paralysis of their lungs or legs. Sister Kenny, an Australian nurse with unorthodox methods for treating polio and preventing paralysis, had come to the United States in 1942 seeking a place to establish a treatment center. Only Minneapolis had responded, giving her $5,000 and a ward at General Hospital. She soon wanted a larger space for her treatment center.

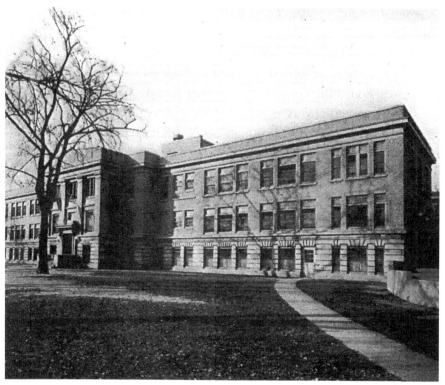

The Lymanhurst. (Courtesy of the Hennepin History Museum)

16

Confrontations and Cures

SISTER KENNY HAD HER EYE on a specific space for her clinic: the old Ly-manhurst building at Eighteenth and Chicago, which was then known as the Minneapolis Public Health Center. Making room for the poliomyelitis cases would mean relocating the tuberculosis clinic, a venereal disease clin-ic, the Variety Heart Clinic, and forty children who were receiving resident treatment at the heart hospital. Negotiations for the space were described as "wrangling," a "controversy," and "petty quarrels" in the daily newspapers. The old Hopewell Hospital, which had been renamed Parkview Sanatorium, was suggested as a site for the polio clinic, but Sister Kenny said Lymanhurst was the only building available that met her requirements.[1]

The Sanatorium Commission offered a solution. Perhaps the existing tuberculosis services, including the diagnostic clinics at Fairview Hospital, University Hospital, and a city clinic at General Hospital could be put to-gether under the direction of Glen Lake Sanatorium. That proposal met with vigorous opposition from several physicians. This consolidation discus-sion, described as a "fight" by a local reporter, had started six years earlier and died out, but the polio-related relocation re-ignited the issue of control over local tuberculosis services.[2]

In August 1942, the Minneapolis board of public welfare approved the Lymanhurst building as the site for Sister Kenny's clinic, and it opened in October. The tuberculosis clinics were moved to remodeled storage space at the General Hospital, but the Variety Heart Clinic and the children in the heart hospital remained at Lymanhurst. Although many members of the board opposed the move, the resident heart patients were eventually relocat-ed to the Glen Lake Children's Building in November 1943, while the clinic remained at Lymanhurst. Other sites offered as alternatives were deemed unsuitable or too expensive to remodel.[3]

Meanwhile, the tuberculosis death rate was increasing. A national report showed more men than women struck by tuberculosis, with the greatest rise in the fifteen to forty-five age group. Dr. Stephen Baxter of the Hennepin County Tuberculosis Association warned that a twenty-five percent increase in the tuberculosis death rate from 1942 to 1943 pointed to the possibility of a shortage of sanatorium beds after the war.[4]

The old problem of inebriation and intractable patients also became a prominent issue in 1942. A Hennepin County grand jury was appointed to investigate the problem of alcoholism at the sanatorium, prompted by complaints made by neighbors. Of special concern was Jack's Tavern. Dr. Mariette agreed that patients were going to the place to drink alcohol and "creating a danger to the public and the patients." Residents of the Glen Lake area opposed renewal of the beer license and it was denied by the Hennepin County commissioners in June 1942.[5]

Denying a license to Jack's Tavern did not solve the problem. Another grand jury investigation in 1944 reported that patients frequently went to Hopkins during their exercise privileges and then returned to the sanatorium intoxicated. No recommendations by the jury seem to have been followed.[6]

In 1945, the board of public welfare asked Minneapolis mayor Hubert Humphrey to appoint a committee to find a solution for "incorrigible patients." Dr. Mariette had requested that a section of the city workhouse be segregated for tuberculous lawbreakers. No solution was implemented, primarily because workhouse personnel refused to be responsible for inmates with tuberculosis.[7]

The end of the war came in sight on May 8, 1945. The day of victory in Europe was celebrated by the Glen Lake dietary department, which served coffee and cookies to the sanatorium employees. *Terrace Topics* noted that it was enjoyed by all, but with restraint in the gaiety. Everyone was still aware that the Pacific war was not yet won.

On August 14, 1945, with the surrender of the Japanese forces, everyone was able to celebrate the end of the war without restraint, but the effects of the war lasted long after the celebrations ended.[8]

Tuberculosis was an issue for the armed forces, just as in World War I. The Minnesota Veterans Hospital near Fort Snelling did not have a special tuberculosis hospital, instead reserving 187 of its 1,000 regular beds for the tuberculous. It was also not equipped to care for female veterans. Glen Lake had admitted its first war veteran in January 1944. She was a member of the WAVES (Women Accepted for Volunteer Emergency Service) who contracted tuberculosis during service.[9]

The VA hospitals in general were earning a bad reputation for care. The nation was alerted to overcrowding and high death rates at the hospitals by Albert Q. Maisel through an article published in *Cosmopolitan* and republished in an April 1945 issue of *Reader's Digest*. Maisel said, "Our disabled veterans are being betrayed by the incompetence, bureaucracy and callousness of the Veterans' Administration." He castigated the administration for unhygienic practices and understaffing, and also accused them of publishing deceptive statistics.

A portion of his article contrasted Minnesota's VA hospital with Glen Lake's operation. The physician-to-patient ratio at the VA was one to fifty-nine, whereas that of Glen Lake was one to forty-one. At the VA in 1944, seventy-eight percent of the veterans with tuberculosis were discharged as having had no benefit from the treatment (including death), while at Glen Lake for the same time period, only twenty-five percent of discharged patients were unimproved or dead.[10] Dr. Josewich from the VA hospital submitted a rebuttal to the *Minneapolis Star-Journal*, calling the article untrue and unfair.[11] Regardless of its accuracy, Maisel's exposé had an immediate effect.

In the December 1945 issue of *Reader's Digest*, Maisel reported that General Omar Bradley had been appointed as the new administrator of Veteran's Affairs and had began to overhaul and modernize their ninety-five hospitals. Bradley's primary goal was to break a cycle of hiring practices that prevented the hospitals from being approved for internships and residencies by the American Medical Association. That in turn hindered them from hiring high-quality physicians. He also created a special services division to oversee private concessionaires who ran unsanitary canteens and stores in the institutions, and he worked with transportation officials to set up priority transportation for ill and wounded veterans.[12] Bradley also encouraged hospitals to negotiate contracts with state and local sanatoriums that were already well-equipped to handle tuberculosis cases.

Dr. Mariette pointed out that welcoming tuberculous war veterans would mean reopening two of the previously closed floors. He warned that caring for veterans properly would be a challenge for the sanatorium if more general duty nurses weren't hired. The contract system also met opposition from veterans' groups. A petition signed by several veterans claimed that Glen Lake's distance from Fort Snelling would bring delays in Veterans' Administration services and deter visitors.[13]

Despite objections, a contract to house up to 125 veterans was signed in May 1946. Under the contract system, most of the VA hospital's tuberculosis patients were transferred to Glen Lake or other county sanatoriums. Female veterans were cared for on contract, too, even if they didn't have tuberculosis.[14]

By 1946, forty veterans were at Glen Lake, and eighty-five more were waiting to be transferred pending the hiring of additional staff. In order to cope with the increased patient load, several patients up on exercise performed simple care duties to help the nurses.

Harold G. "Snuff" Kurvers was one of the veterans taking the cure at Glen Lake. Kurvers survived the Bataan Death March and was in a prison camp until August 1945. He returned to the U.S. but spent most of 1946 at the sanatorium, recovering from tuberculosis. He married Dorothy at Glen Lake in January, and she lived with his aunt in Hopkins so she could be close enough to visit every day.[15]

Members of various rural Hennepin County American Legion organizations came to Glen Lake to visit the veterans there. They brought candy, t-shirts, pajamas, and other items in an attempt to thank those who were now suffering because of their military service. They also held bedside initiation ceremonies so veterans could become Legion members.[16]

Some veterans proved to be difficult patients who exhibited both serious behavioral problems not well understood at the time and simple high spirits from surviving the war. Medical staff commented on how they pushed back on the rules by going to Hopkins without leave, playing cards whenever they pleased, and having contraband radios. Cars were a special point of contention, with veterans described as being belligerent when asked to remove their cars from the campus. One doctor suggested letting air out of tires or taking off the wheels, solutions that weren't implemented. Dr. Mariette instead reminded the veterans that Glen Lake was a civilian hospital, and they had to abide by the same rules as the other patients.[17]

Glen Lake also welcomed other people whose lives or health had been disrupted by the war.

May Tanaka was diagnosed as having an active case of tuberculosis while in a Japanese internment camp in Arizona. She spent a year in the camp's hospital, and her family moved to Minnesota after their release. Her TB reactivated and she underwent rib removals at Glen Lake to collapse her lung."[18]

Fumi Tanamachi and her husband, Masao, came to Minnesota from California when he was assigned to the Army's Military Intelligence Service Language School at Fort Snelling. Masao was one of 6,000 Japanese citizens trained in Minnesota to serve as translators and code breakers for the Army. Fumi was diagnosed with tuberculosis. She came to Glen Lake for treatment, was discharged, and lived to age sixty-eight.[19]

Fumio Shishino was not so fortunate. His family was taken first to the Santa Anita racetrack in California, where they lived in horse stalls, and then they were transported by train to Gila River Relocation Center in Arizona. In 1943, Fumio's son obtained a job at a resort in northern Minnesota, and he was able to arrange for the rest of the family to follow. In January 1946, Fumio was admitted to Glen Lake, where he died in March.[20]

Dr. Shih Hao Tsai came to the United States in 1947 in order to obtain more training in tuberculosis treatment. His mother's death from TB in the 1930s gave him a personal interest in the disease. Tsai had two offers of employment—one from a hospital in New York with no pay and another from Dr. Mariette for eighty dollars per month for a year. He chose Minnesota. After World War II, China's civil war resumed and the communist People's Republic of China took over the mainland. Tsai's wife and father told him not to come home. Because Tsai couldn't get a license to practice medicine as a non-citizen, he was appointed to a fellowship, which was continued until he achieved citizenship. His wife, Yukee (Ruby), arrived in 1949 and worked briefly at Glen Lake as a nurse's aide.[21]

Dr. Wen (Wayne) Yue, from Putian, China, also came to Minnesota to work at Glen Lake. He, too, intended to return home after a period of study but remained in the United States because of political unrest. When the sanatorium closed, Tsai decided to specialize in radiology, while Yue chose anesthesiology. Both co-authored several TB-related articles in medical journals and worked at the Veterans' Hospital later in their careers.[22]

The search for a cure for tuberculosis continued throughout the war and actually benefitted from medical advances prompted by battlefield injuries.

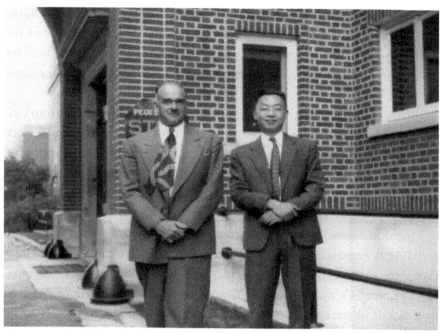

Tsai. (Courtesy of the Tsai family)

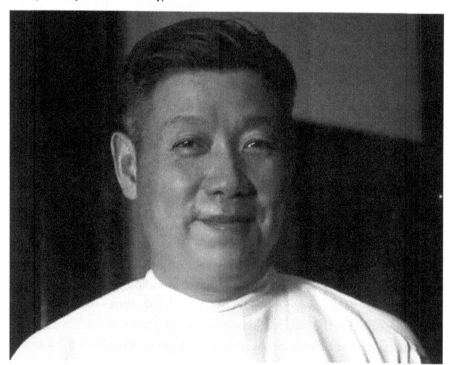

Yue. (Courtesy of the Yue family)

Because of Glen Lake's association with the Mayo Clinic, patients with far-advanced tuberculosis were given the opportunity to participate in clinical drug trials. A one-year project had begun in June 1941 to test a sulfone drug, Promin, provided by Parke-Davis and Company. Because so little was known about these drugs, patients participating were generally hopeless cases, chronic cases, or they had renal tuberculosis.

Glen Lake, Mayo Clinic, and Mineral Springs together were considered one testing site. The others were Metropolitan Life Insurance Company in McGregor Sanatorium, New York, and the William Maybury Sanatorium near Detroit, Michigan.[23] The drug was moderately successful with leprosy, which is also caused by a mycobacteria, but it was not very effective with TB. In 1944, doctors H. Corwin Hinshaw and William Feldman were featured in a magazine article about a newer version of the sulfone drug. *Collier's* hailed it as a cure, and the two doctors took the editors to task for giving the public a mistaken impression.[24]

In April 1944, a female patient who had been at Glen Lake since 1936 began participation in a clinical drug trial for Diasone. A similar trial was being administered by doctors Karl Pfuetze and Marjorie Pyle at the nearby

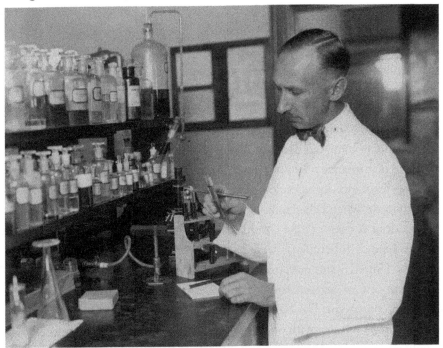

Laboratory. (Courtesy of the Hennepin History Museum)

Mineral Springs sanatorium in Cannon Falls. The drug had also been tested in Illinois by Dr. Charles Petter, a former senior resident at Glen Lake. It had seemed effective there, but the Minnesota results were disappointing. Many of the patients were unable to continue the medication because of toxic side effects. Glen Lake's patient died in 1945.[25]

At Mayo Clinic in Rochester, Feldman and Hinshaw received a small amount of streptomycin from Dr. Selman Waksman and his laboratory assistant, Albert Schatz, who worked at Rutgers University. Experiments were performed at Mayo with four guinea pigs in the fall of 1944. Hinshaw and Feldman autopsied the guinea pigs, and results indicated that streptomycin could suppress tuberculosis. They repeated the tests and saw the same results. They had a limited supply of the drug, and they considered using some of it on a tuberculous patient whose prognosis was grim.[26]

Patricia Thomas was a patient in Mineral Springs who was diagnosed with far-advanced tuberculosis in her right lung. A phrenic nerve crush and four stages of thoracoplastic surgery had little effect, and her tuberculosis spread to the left lung. She was selected as an appropriate patient on which to test streptomycin because her prognosis was imminent death. On November 20, 1944, she received the first dose. She began to improve and the streptomycin was discontinued on April 7, 1945.[27]

Despite the apparent success with Patricia Thomas, Dr. Hinshaw warned that many problems were yet to be solved in its use. It didn't seem to destroy the tuberculosis but instead held the bacilli in check so that the body was better equipped to self-heal. Further study was needed on its effect on tuberculosis of the bones and joints, skin, and internal organs. Known drawbacks included its potential to damage the vestibulocochlear nerve and cause deafness and disturbance of equilibrium. He also warned about the development of drug resistance in tubercle bacilli. Hinshaw asked doctors to avoid using streptomycin when other treatments worked, because to inadvertently produce a drug-resistant strain would make streptomycin ineffective if a more serious type of tuberculosis were to develop.[28]

The United States government also conducted tests on new drugs. Glen Lake was one of six sanatoria in the country that took part in a drug trial for streptomycin. Dr. Sumner Cohen went to Washington, D.C., every three months to meet with other doctors working on the same project. They would evaluate the progress of patients taking the drug, comparing those on

Regimen I, II, or III. Researchers found that streptomycin could cure meningitis in children. It was worth the risk of side effects, including deafness, because tuberculosis meningitis in children was always fatal.[29]

One of the drugs tested showed promise for people with mental health issues, but it didn't have any effect on tuberculosis. Another of the drugs tested in at Glen Lake in 1945 was Pyricidin, for which isoniazid is the generic name. Dr. Mariette cautioned the medical staff that there was to be no publicity about the testing. That drug proved to have value, and was used in combination with other drugs for treatment of tuberculosis.[30]

Some drugs were also tested at Anoka State Hospital, and about thirty-five patients from Glen Lake participated in a drug trial there. Fred Maurer, who started working at the sanatorium in 1945 as a driver, would transport the patients to Anoka every few weeks, where they would be evaluated. Maurer recalled the time as an exciting era. "I enjoyed my work so much I would have worked for free. It was the beginning of the eradication of TB. You hoped to work yourself out of a job because you wanted TB to be cured."[31]

By 1947, streptomycin's efficacy had been established, and it was available in limited quantities for use at Glen Lake, especially for veterans through continuing federal research. Dr. Cohen represented Glen Lake at a Veterans'

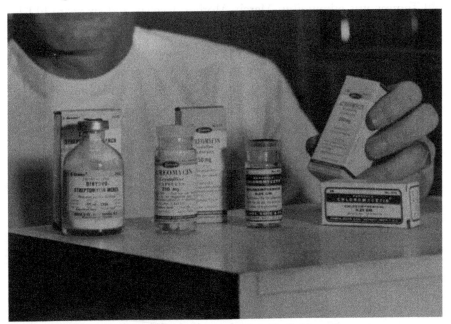

Drugs. (Courtesy of the University of Minnesota-Duluth Martin Library))

Administration streptomycin conference in Atlanta, being one of only two non-federal hospitals participating.

Nurse Deloise Anderson Clair remembered that there was a lot of paper work and a lot of pills involved in those drug trials. Most of the patients got twenty-four pills a day, plus about four niacin pills and whatever other medications they were getting. The strep nurse wore gloves, gown, and hat to keep from getting sensitized to the streptomycin.[32]

Tragically, only those patients who were in a drug trial or were able to personally pay for streptomycin received it. The drug was expensive to administer, at a cost of $400 per patient (equivalent to about $4,400 in 2016). The Hennepin County Tuberculosis Association gave a $10,000 grant of Christmas seals funds to Glen Lake at the beginning of 1947 to cover streptomycin purchases, and that was quickly exhausted. The association added another $2,600 to the fund in November.[33]

Families touched by tuberculosis were experiencing better outcomes thanks to streptomycin. For example, all five members of one family were at Glen Lake. Baby Jimmy Grose had contracted tuberculosis meningitis and lived for only three months in 1946. His father, Clarence Grose, and oldest sister, Elaine, were brought to the sanitorium on New Year's Eve. Two-year-old Tommy was admitted in March. Mother, Evelyn, and six-year-old Clareen joined them in August.[34] Elaine had tuberculosis meningitis, so she was moved from the Children's Building to the main building. After four months of streptomycin therapy provided by Christmas seal funds, she was able to go back to the Children's Building. In March 1948, she went home with her mother and then returned to attend the summer camp.[35]

Jimmie Olson, age six, also escaped certain death thanks to streptomycin. A patient at Glen Lake with his mother since he was almost two years old, he was about ready to be sent home when he fell into a semi-coma with tuberculosis meningitis. He was immediately put on double shots of streptomycin, paid for in part by a fundraising effort launched by his father. Veterans of Foreign Wars posts and their auxiliaries supported the entire course of treatment, which cost nearly $1,000.[36]

Not all applications of the drug were successful. A young Japanese boy interned in the camps in California had tuberculosis of the kidney. The diseased kidney was removed, and he relocated to Minnesota with his family. When they arrived, it was discovered that he had far-advanced tuberculosis in the remaining kidney. The Heffelfingers, a wealthy family from Minneapolis, provided streptomycin for him—several shots a day—but he eventually died. Nurse Phyllis Burns, who gave him his first shot, said, "It was very hard to lose one like that."[37]

By 1948, the price of streptomycin dropped due to increased and improved production. Dosages became more precise and effective, but the germs had become more effective, too, and developed resistance to the drug. Initial trials with another drug, Para Aminosalicylic (PAS) acid, proved to be as successful as those with streptomycin, but those patients were also developing drug-resistant germs. The British Medical Council launched a trial combining streptomycin and PAS. The same combined investigational trials began in the U.S. Veterans' Administration hospitals and its contract institutions, including Glen Lake.[38,39]

Both Wayne Engstrom and his brother Robert received streptomycin injections. Wayne had streptomycin shots two times a week for a short period of time, and they made him afraid of needles. Robert had a more advanced case of tuberculosis, so he needed strong doses. It was injected with a needle so long that he wouldn't look at it. The nurse came in the morning to give the shot. What hurt more than the actual puncture was how it expanded the tissue it went into. It seemed, to him, to take forever to get the syringe emptied. It expanded so much that he felt like he had a golf ball in his buttocks. "That was a painful type of medication," he said.

The Engstroms' father was the first from the family to enter the sanatorium and was probably the source of infection for the children. He was on strict bed for about three years, had several surgeries, and spent almost ten years there. Their sister Nancy, a third-grader, was in the Children's Building. After the father's discharge from the sanatorium, he moved to northern Minnesota and gave his house to Wayne with the understanding that he would take care of the younger children, which he did.[40]

Chemotherapy did not eliminate the need for surgical intervention, either. Although the bacilli were conquered, the body sometimes needed assistance to heal. In 1949, 259 stages were performed on ninety-nine patients.[41] New forms of anesthesia made it possible to do more extensive surgery when it was necessary to removed diseased portions of lungs. Any operation on diseased lungs could spread TB bacteria into the pleural cavity, and that would produce an infection called empyema. The infection could be worse for the patient than the condition for which the surgery was attempted. When patients were given anti-TB drugs for a period of six months before the surgery, there would be fewer complications from infections. New surgical methods allowed doctors to excise only the affected wedges of a lung, down to a piece the size of a golf ball or less.[42]

By 1946, Glen Lake had changed dramatically from the three-building cottage sanatorium of thirty years before. The triune treatment of rest, good food, and fresh air had evolved into complex surgeries and chemical interventions. Patients were not merely kept entertained, but they were provided opportunities for education and training that fitted them for occupations some had never hoped to attain. The campus itself, which once had existed in a near-empty expanse of woods and pastures, now had many neighbors.

Along with losing physical isolation, Glen Lake's administration was also losing the autonomy it enjoyed by having highly respected and influential men governing its operation through long service on the sanatorium commission. Edward Gale, an original member, died in September 1943, a year after his retirement from the commission. Joseph Kingman served from 1916 to 1942. Dr. Marx White had served from 1919 to 1937, taken a three-year break, and returned in 1940. The other two positions had been filled for brief periods by several people, including Dr. Francis E. Harrington, L.G. Nygren, W.F. Kunze, Lois M. Fraser, and Raymond Ryti.

With the exception of Dr. Harrington, a physician at Glen Lake in the 1920s, the commissioners seemed to have relatively little experience in tuberculosis treatment or in hospital administration. Their oversight duties seem to have lapsed into reactive approvals to Mariette's proposals. When steady hands were needed to guide the sanatorium through dramatic changes in treatment, financial crises, and political squabbles, the commissioners were conspicuously absent from the public debates. Dr. Mariette became the sanatorium representative most often quoted in the newspapers.

Some of the political conflict over control of tuberculosis services eased in 1945, when a new Hennepin County Public Health Center opened at 240 South Fourth Street, Minneapolis. It housed the chest clinic once operated at Fairview Hospital by Glen Lake and the Hennepin County Tuberculosis Association, the tuberculosis treatment (pneumothorax) clinic once operated at the University of Minnesota by Glen Lake, the clinics of the Minneapolis Health Department, the public health nursing staff of the Minneapolis

Health Department, and the Glen Lake Outpatient Department office formerly operating out of the sanatorium.[43]

Although the hospital for children with rheumatic fever was housed at Glen Lake, the Variety Club clinic was still co-located with the Kenny Institute in the old Lymanhurst building. In November 1945, the institute requested that the board of public welfare remove the heart clinic, even though there was a five-year space agreement. The *Star Journal* reported that this was accompanied by a threat from Sister Kenny to leave Minneapolis if the request wasn't approved.[44]

Although not directly related, the arrival of Sister Kenny and the subsequent "turf wars" over the clinics marked a change in the relationship between the Minneapolis community and the Glen Lake Sanatorium. Newspaper coverage of the sanatorium up to this point had consisted mostly of human interest stories that portrayed the institution and its governance in a favorable light. Although various medical organizations and political factions had disagreed in private, those differences had simmered quietly until 1942. Once the clinic controversy gained placement on the front pages of newspapers, the sanatorium's long honeymoon period with the press was over.

17

Financial Crisis

THERE'S A SAYING THAT CLAIMS if you want something done, you get a busy person to do it. For years, that saying held true for Glen Lake Sanatorium, too. Under Dr. Mariette's leadership and with an able staff, the sanatorium had set upon a path of continual improvement in cooperation with many local and national organizations. Sometimes a busy person reaches a point of being overtaxed, and a breakdown occurs. Coping with war-related shortages and the distractions of additional responsibilities seems to have brought Glen Lake and Dr. Mariette to a sort of tipping point, too.

A series of circumstances, most of them beyond the control of Glen Lake's administration, created another financial crisis. In December 1946, Dr. Mariette reported that Glen Lake would have a deficit of $103,050 and would probably end 1947 in the red, too, if the mill tax levy wasn't raised. Dr. Myers, professor at the University of Minnesota, said publicly that maintaining "a $3,000,000 sanatorium costing $750,000 a year to operate is absurd." He believed that with the new methods of diagnosis and treatment, tuberculosis could be eradicated by 1966.[1] His statement echoed the changing attitude of many taxpayers, who thought tuberculosis was no longer a major threat. There was news of a cure, and it seemed wasteful to pour money into supporting a large specialized hospital.

Dr. Mariette's rebuttal pointed out that operating expenses could not be pared any further without affecting essential services. Mariette also predicted that up to 500 additional TB cases might be identified during an upcoming county-wide X-ray survey, and extra beds and nurses would be needed. The institution could not utilize 104 existing beds without additional staffing. He also believed that the institution was worth the investment, because it could serve other purposes after TB was conquered. He said, "No money spent on building facilities here can ever be considered wasted. The plant is easily adaptable to other hospital purposes should the decline in TB leave it vacant." He also pointed out the lack of a hospital in the western part of the county and said the sanatorium was "a building admirably suited for a general hospital for rural Hennepin County—circumstances, the medical profession, and the politicians willing."[2,3,4]

Part of the funding crisis originated in previous sessions of the state legislature when all other county sanatoriums were allowed to raise their mill rate limitation for funding. Because Glen Lake was operating in the black at the time, it did not receive approval to raise additional funds through taxation. Also, the change to a forty-hour work week meant that 167 additional employees were needed to cover the hours previously worked by people working in excess of fifty hours a week.[5]

An article in *The Spectator* asked, "What's Glen Lake Worth?" and that question was repeated in many editorials. Former patient Jane Eads Watson responded with a letter to the editor, saying that hope and salvation lie in the magic words, "Glen Lake." Helen Quinn Cooke also wrote to support additional funding. Six years after spending time there as a patient, she reported herself to be not only holding her own, but raising a young daughter as well.[6]

In February 1947, three members of the legislature who represented the county requested that a state public examiner look at Glen Lake's finances. They called Glen Lake's business management inefficient, and claimed that the per capita cost was greatly in excess of costs for similar operations. The examiner, Richard Golling, later met with the Hennepin County senate delegation, which decided there had been no irregularities in the handling of funds.[7]

Also, no suspicion or blame was attributed to Walter Lundahl, who had been the business manager at Glen Lake since 1919. Facing what was certain to become a political scuffle, however, he resigned his position and became a purchaser at Aslesen Company in Minneapolis.[8]

Added to the pressure of the audit was a request by the Hennepin County commissioners that the legislature abolish the sanatorium commission and give control to the county. Commissioner George Matthews pointed out that the county board had jurisdiction over all other county-funded institutions, and that the sanatorium commission members did not seem to have ample time to check on all of the items required. The legislature did not act on that request.[9] Funding bills were introduced, however, and the legislature allowed a levy increase. Hennepin County was allowed to make a transfer of funds from general revenue to the sanatorium fund. It was hoped the infusion of $150,000 into Glen Lake's budget would stabilize its finances until a levy increase could take effect the following year.[10]

The transfer of funds helped to pay the immediate outstanding bills, but changes still needed to be made immediately to lessen demands on the nursing staff. Visiting hours were restricted to three afternoons a week, and other measures were taken to allow for new patients to be admitted and cared for in the existing beds. Two strategies were drastic and unpopular:[11]

(1) Approximately forty patients from other counties who had come to Glen Lake for surgery or special care were ordered back to their home sanatorium. In the long run, this action led to less income because it decreased non-resident revenue by nearly $400 per day.

(2) War veterans who were not residents of the county had to leave, freeing up forty-eight beds. This decision was questioned and criticized in local newspapers.

In addition, patients who had recovered from tuberculosis but were being treated for another condition were sent to other hospitals. Others were readied for discharge four months earlier than usual using a revised privilege and exercise plan. Some staffing relief was obtained by offering higher salaries to nurses and attracting a few new hires. A vacant floor was reopened and the waiting list was whittled down to only twelve applicants.[12]

Meanwhile, Mariette's earlier prediction about the county-wide TB survey proved to be correct. In addition to the Hennepin County screening, the 1947 legislature provided the Department of Health with funding for mobile X-ray units, which traveled throughout the state and offered free chest X-rays to all citizens. By 1948, 509,602 persons had been screened for TB. Glen Lake experienced a sudden influx of applications and twenty-seven people were added to the waiting list.[13,14]

The sanatorium's problems went beyond staffing costs and daily operations, though. The aging pasteurization plant didn't pass inspection, which meant purchasing bottled milk until it was repaired. The administration building had not been updated since construction in 1921, and it needed upgrades to meet new fire and patient-care standards. Mariette estimated it would cost approximately $458,216 to make all the improvements.[15]

The nursing shortage continued, however, and Glen Lake again turned to importing nurses as a partial solution. This time, assistance came from thirteen displaced persons from Latvia, Lithuania, and Estonia who were cleared to work as practical nurses at the sanatorium. Most of them had been in Russian or German concentration camps and were screened by the federal government for health issues and political affiliation. The first two nurses arrived in February 1948 and were sponsored by Lutheran Social Services' resettlement agency and the Church World Service of the National Council of Churches of Christ.[16]

Displaced persons were mostly assigned to work as orderlies and ward maids because most of them barely spoke English.[17]

Edita Vabalaite, one of the first nurses to arrive, was quickly wooed by a former Lithuanian newspaper correspondent, Arejas Vitkauskas, who was looking for a secretary who could speak his language. They married within a month, and she moved to New York.[18]

Another displaced person from Latvia who arrived at Glen Lake was Dr. Erich Buss, who worked there until he could pass state examinations for licensure. Dr. Buss later married Velta Rozentals, a Latvian nurse who came to the U.S. during the war and also worked at Glen Lake.[19]

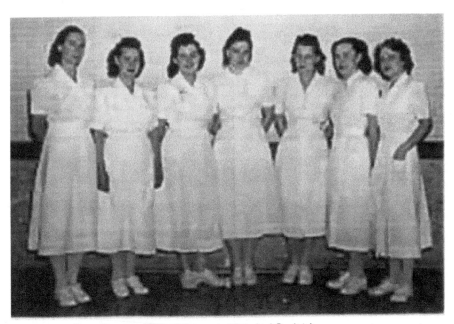

Displaced nurses. (Courtesy of the Minnesota Historical Society)

Even with the economizing strategies and the new employees, the sanatorium ended 1948 with a $153,605 deficit.

Not everything was bad news, though. Despite the administrative difficulties, life went on much as usual within the sanatorium.

Delores Autey, who in 1942 set a national juvenile skating record in the 220-yard dash, entered Glen Lake in 1945. By the time her doctor gave her the all clear to return to skating, Delores had discovered some new talents, as editor of *Terrace Topics* and program director and announcer on KNUT. The gender barrier at KNUT had been broken in 1942, when patients Margaret Nickle and Shirley MacDougall aired a "Classical Hour" program.[20,21]

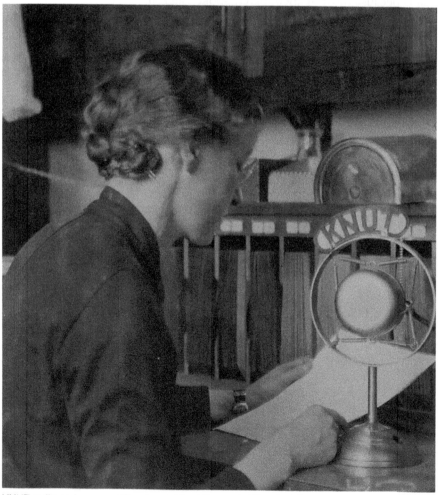

KNUT radio and women. (Courtesy of the Minnesota Historical Society)

Virgil Israelson, who had been in the Children's Building as a child, returned as a teenager. He had come as a three-year-old in 1939 with tuberculosis in his hip. After surgery to fuse it, he was in a body cast from his chest down his right leg. That was later adjusted to be on his leg only, but the surgery and immobilization for three years left him with his right leg shorter than the other. He was about ten years old when he left, but had been able to enjoy some of the adventures that living with other children could offer. He especially enjoyed it when Frank Swan was the orderly on duty, because he sang while he worked.

When Israelson returned in 1949, it was with a case of bacterial meningitis. He endured a series of spinal tests and streptomycin shots. He also was old enough to miss his friends, because as a teenager in the main building, he had few roommates his own age. Once, one of the older men gave him some money and asked him to buy some Aqua Velva aftershave for him at the sanatorium store. When he returned with the purchase, the man drank the aftershave and Israelson got scolded for buying it for him. Because paralysis set in, his second stay was thirty months long. Once he felt better, he could stand by the bed and then he learned to walk again by pushing a chair.[22]

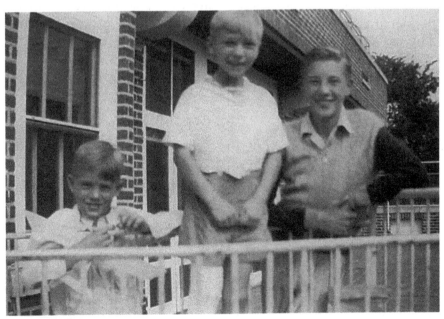

Israelson. (Courtesy of the Israelson family)

Physicians continued to come from other states and countries to study Minnesota's approach to tuberculosis control. A public health training course brought Dr. McDermid from Rochester, New York; Dr. Holm from Copenhagen, Denmark; and Dr. Kurland, from Baltimore, Maryland, to Glen Lake.[23] Dr. Paulo Baptista arrived from Brazil to study TB treatment and chest surgery.[24] The physicians and administrative staff posed for a photo to send as a greeting to the colleagues who had visited the sanatorium.

The cheer committee from the Shriners paid their usual Christmas visit to the sanatorium in 1945. Patients who were up on exercise continued to help out where needed. The first post-war Christmas season saw the post office sending out and receiving more than forty mailbags of packages. Six patients played "postman" and used wheelchairs as carts to make rounds to pick up and deliver letters and packages. The official postmaster, James Collins, was an ex-patient, as was the clerk, Floyd Nelson.[25]

A fire in 1946 fortunately caused no harm to any patients and only superficial damage to the auditorium. Some floor waxing was being done near the stage, and the small explosion and fire were blamed on the spontaneous combustion of cloths used in that process. It did curtail movie nights for a while, though.[26]

Also in 1946, a particularly severe outbreak of polio touched Minnesota. One out of every 2,114 Minnesotans had reportedly been infected with the virus, and the annual state fair was cancelled. This was a disappointment to

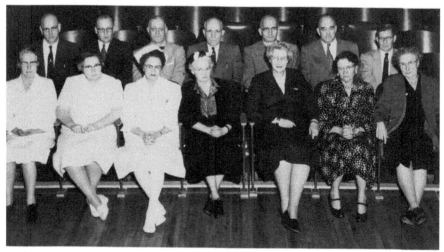

Medical and administrative staff. (Courtesy of the Minnesota Historical Society)

Glen Lake's occupational therapy patients, who looked forward to exhibiting in the Women's Building. They had missed the opportunity in 1945, too, when federal transportation restrictions closed the fair.[27]

Articles made by the Glen Lake patients reappeared at the state fair in 1947. Sanatorium patients had always competed in a special category created for them, but that year they were allowed for the first time to join the general public in the women's division. They proved their skills by capturing several first prizes. One of the winners was Lynn Brewster, a male World War II veteran who won a blue ribbon for his knitted socks. Two women who produced nearly identical linen tablecloths with Italian hemstitching, one blue and one yellow, won sweepstake and second prize. The patients also had a good year in 1948, winning thirty first prizes and two sweepstakes awards.[28]

Dr. Mariette was in demand as a speaker, both locally and nationally. In September 1946, he addressed the Mississippi Valley Trudeau Society in Chicago as its president, and he read a paper at the American Hospital Association in Philadelphia. In 1947, he replaced Dr. Baxter as president of the Hennepin County Tuberculosis Association, and in June he attended the annual convention of the National Tuberculosis Association in San Francisco. He made stops at sanatoriums in Colorado on his way back home.

The problem of incorrigible and inebriated patients continued and the complaints from neighbors intensified. The sanatorium still operated under the commitment procedure of 1913. In the past, some offenders could be hauled off to the county jail, but new state health regulations did not allow the sheriff to house people with communicable diseases. Deputies could go out to Glen Lake to try to quiet down an inebriated patient, but it was left up to the nurses and doctors to make them stay there. In spite of several requests to the legislature over the years, no special institution or policy had been established for handling difficult patients.

When asked why Glen Lake didn't institute harsh measures to prevent drinking and going to bars, Dr. Mariette replied that the sanatorium did not search visitors and "nor do we prevent patients who are able from walking around. The place is not a penal institution."[29]

There continued to be a stigma attached to having had tuberculosis. Sometimes, patients asked for leave to go home, and then the patients' family would call the sanatorium and ask why they were allowed to do that. It was an embarrassing situation for the patient, so a new policy stipulated that a social worker should call the family first to confirm their willingness to have a TB patient visit them.[30]

Glen Lake continued its participation in drug trials. Its resident population of people with tuberculosis who were also alcoholics caught the attention of a Canadian pharmaceutical company, Ayerst, McKenna & Harrison, Ltd. They contacted the sanatorium in May, offering participation in a research study for Antabuse, a drug to treat chronic alcoholism. Glen Lake accepted and would have been the only tuberculosis sanatorium participating, but the physicians decided they didn't have time to do a study not related to TB, and later declined.[31]

The financial crisis was another issue that would not go away. In spite of the tax levies and the transfer of $150,000, the state public examiner announced in July 1949 that Glen Lake finished 1948 with a deficit of $123,390.[32]

One could speculate that it was not a coincidence that Dr. Mariette suffered a cerebral hemorrhage in August 1949 at age sixty-one. Since 1916, Mariette had served as both medical director and superintendent, and the past few years had seen the sanatorium lurch from one challenge to another. Hindsight can say that, as Glen Lake grew, a division of duties may have benefitted both the sanatorium and his health. In addition, while coping with the turnover of sanatorium commissioners during the turbulent years of the 1940s, he also often navigated a political arena that was their responsibility.

Just days after his stroke, the legislature authorized a $4.75 million levy allowing the sanatorium to raise more than $1,000,000 and have a balanced budget in the coming year. The news came to Mariette at Eitel Hospital in Minneapolis, where his wife reported that he was "doing very nicely." In reality, the effects of the stroke were severe, and he would require twenty-four-hour nursing care for the remainder of his life.[33,34]

Mariette resigned as superintendent of Glen Lake on September 8, 1949, with an effective date of November 1. Tributes in the local newspapers acknowledged the doctor's thirty-three years of service at the sanatorium and in the community as a strong advocate for innovation in medical treatments and vocational education. He had served longer as a sanatorium superintendent than any other person in Minnesota. Special mention was given to his early vision of the sanatorium as a conventional hospital rather than the cottage-type institution popular at the time. The editor of *Oak Leaves*, Glen Lake's employee newsletter, said, "If each of us might accomplish for humanity half of what Dr. Mariette has done in those thirty-three years, we might look upon our lives as indeed more than worthwhile."[35]

Dr. Peter Mattill, a long-time physician at Glen Lake, was appointed acting superintendent. He had himself contracted tuberculosis and was briefly at Nopeming Sanatorium before arriving at Glen Lake in 1924. For a long time he wrote a regular column for *Terrace Topics*, and he had served as assistant superintendent since 1938. He and his family resided in one of the three doctors' houses on campus.

Dr. Russell Frost assumed superintendent duties in February 1950. He had worked at Glen Lake briefly in 1928 and then was in charge of Buena Vista Sanatorium in Wabasha until 1939. He spent three years as head of the G.B. Cooley Sanatorium in West Monroe, Louisiana. In 1942, he returned to Minnesota to be the chief of the tuberculosis service at Fort Snelling. By accepting the position at Glen Lake, he became responsible for a sanatorium whose obsolescence was on the horizon.[36]

Dr. J. Arthur Myers published his book, *Invited and Conquered*, in 1949. It chronicled one hundred years of anti-tuberculosis efforts in Minnesota, and the title reflected everyone's optimistic response to news about the healing powers of streptomycin. Tuberculosis was no longer one of the ten leading causes of death for Minnesotans. The dreaded scourge that had menaced mankind for centuries was on the brink of being controlled.[37]

18

Transitions

B OB DYLAN DIDN'T RELEASE THE ALBUM *The Times They Are a-Changin'* until
1964, but the song certainly fits the decade of the 1950s and the rapid
changes in tuberculosis treatment and control.

About the only thing that didn't change at the sanatorium was childbirth.
On New Year's Day 1950, Mrs. Yow Hom saw her baby girl for the first time,
six weeks after she was born. Becky was the first baby of Chinese ancestry
born at Glen Lake and, following the old pattern, would be seeing her mother every three weeks until they were discharged.[1]

KNUT radio station had changed to WGLS, and its format included a
"Behind the Doors" program that interviewed both sanatorium employees
and people from the community. The 1950 lineup included Dr. Frost, the
dietary department, Clellan Card from WCCO's TV show *Axel and His Dog*,
WCCO radio announcer Bob DeHaven, and *Minneapolis Tribune* columnist
George Grimm.[2]

The ban against individual radios was slowly loosening. Men living in the
East Cottage could have their own radios, as long as they were turned off
at 10:00 p.m. Women in the West Cottage requested the same privilege. A
black-and-white television set was placed in a common lounge in the main
building.[3]

The facility itself was changing. The power plant converted from coal
to gas and oil, and the sanatorium purchased electricity from Northern State
Power Company instead of using coal to generate it on campus. The area
around Glen Lake was changing, too. Streetcar service to Glen Lake and
beyond was being converted to buses. Minnetonka Township had shrunk in
size as portions were annexed by neighboring Wayzata, Hopkins, Deephav-

en, and Woodland, but it had grown significantly in population. It counted 12,000 residents in the 1950 census.

That summer was the last for the children's camp at Birch Island Lake. The odds were now in favor of successful recoveries, and that was especially true among children. Many of the early cases in the Children's Building had been orthopedic due to bovine tuberculosis. The proliferation of pasteurized milk made that infection rare. Glen Lake's Children's Building still had young patients, but most were children of adult patients or meningitis sufferers responding to streptomycin.[4]

The campus mourned when news came that Dr. Mariette died on October 29, 1950. Services at were held at Plymouth Congregational Church with interment at Lakewood Cemetery in Minneapolis. An E.S. Mariette Scholarship for Tuberculosis was established at University of Minnesota in his memory. A fund was also set up to commission an oil painting to be done from photos of the doctor. When completed, it hung in the building's main lobby for many years.[5]

In December, the physicians began a Merck & Co. study comparing streptomycin to dihydrostreptomycin, a similar antibacterial drug. Another study was for TB-1 or Tibione, a drug from Schenley Laboratories in New York. Because there was a possibility of liver damage, TB-1 was given only to cases not helped by streptomycin.[6]

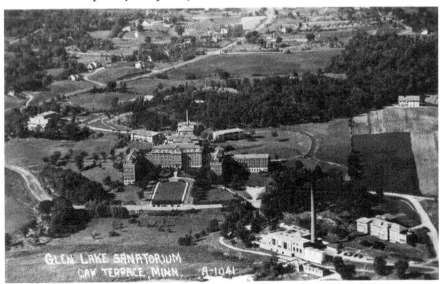

Aerial of campus. (Courtesy of the Minnesota Historical Society)

The medical staff also initiated an Alcoholics Anonymous group for patients. Disruptive patients were increasing in number. Tuberculosis law Chapter 314 was passed in 1951 to give county boards authority to commit a person infected with tuberculosis on the basis of a health officer's report, but members of the Minnesota Board of Health were not optimistic about its usefulness. This new law simplified the commitment procedure, but made no assignment for where the committed patients should go. Without locks and bars at the sanatoriums, it simply would not work for them.

The Anoka State Hospital staff objected to their facility being used as a jail. The St. Cloud Reformatory wasn't suitable for caring for tuberculous patients, and the State Sanatorium staff had threatened to quit if they had to take care of incorrigibles.[7] At one time, the Glen Lake night watchman and the power plant engineer were deputized to incarcerate incorrigible patients, but because they never received any training, the county sheriff refused to work with them.[8]

Dr. Frost explained the problem at Glen Lake:

> Our present need is for twenty locked ward cells. Actually, we have only one four-bed locked ward. We are also using four single locked rooms which are not escape proof. The sanatorium has the right to confiscate liquor when found and does so. While Glen Lake technically has legal authority "to place and confine such patients in quarters apart from other patients," it lacks facilities and personnel to handle the problem. In a sense, the passage of the bill has operated as a handicap to a local solution of the problem because when county authorities are approached, they can justifiably say that the State has assumed the responsibility.[9]

Glen Lake no longer served as a contract hospital for the state mental institutions or for the Veterans' Administration Hospital. In 1952, a building opened at Anoka State Hospital specifically to serve tuberculous mentally ill patients from the state hospitals. It was named the Burns Memorial Building in honor of Dr. Herbert A. Burns, who was with the state Board of Health from 1912 to 1920. As superintendent of the State Sanatorium from 1929 to 1942, he employed an epidemiologist to trace the path of tuberculosis infection to and from the patients. As chief of the state's tuberculosis control unit from 1942, he conducted a study among prison inmates and residents of the state mental hospitals.

In 1952, another polio epidemic struck Hennepin County, and General Hospital wanted to send eleven of their tuberculosis patients to Glen Lake so they could make room for polio victims. The sanatorium was able to take only six because of continued staffing problems.[10]

Also in 1952, a special part of the sanatorium life disappeared when *Terrace Topics* ceased publication in the magazine format. Occasional issues were printed in newsletter format but it no longer measured up to the professionally written and edited publication of the 1930s and '40s.

One of the many sanatorium romances played out on national TV when Emil Grinvalds, a patient from Latvia, married nurse Donna Woods on the program *Queen for a Day*. They received household goods and a free honeymoon. Emil attended Dunwoody Institute after his discharge.[11]

Glen Lake's tradition of teaching and educating continued into the 1950s. Gilbert Lange took advantage of the training system. He had not finished high school as a teenager, but as a former TB patient he could not continue his job as a welder. Lange finished school at Glen Lake and then studied electronics at Dunwoody for two years. He worked in that field until he retired.[12]

The medical records department was instructing other institutions on the challenges of and solutions for setting up medical record libraries in long-term care institutions. Helen Bender's tutoring included correspondence to hospitals in Edmonton, Alberta, Canada; Harlingen, Texas; Oak Forest, Illinois; and Seattle, Washington.[13]

Chemotherapy continued to be augmented by surgery, with 175 pulmonary resections performed at Glen Lake in 1953. Carol Anderson benefitted from both. She was in nurses' training at St. Olaf College when she found out that she had tuberculosis. It was probably contracted from her mother, who died at Nopeming Sanatorium when Carol was ten years old. Her mother also lost two brothers to the disease. Because Anderson's home was in Fergus Falls, she was admitted to Ah-gwah-ching. After she had been there for about four months, she was brought to Glen Lake, where Dr. Kinsella performed surgery to remove a segment of a lung section. Anderson also received streptomycin three times a week, as an injection in the buttocks, and took about a tablespoon of para-aminosalicylic acid (PAS) orally. PAS was administered as a dry powder that looked like brown grain or as a liquid solution. It tasted awful and caused nausea and diarrhea, but the combination of drugs reduced the risk of streptomycin-resistant tubercle bacilli.[14,15]

More visitors came to study and observe. Among them were Dr. Knus Buhl from Denmark; Dr. F.R. Bringos from Obregon, Sonora, Mexico; Mr. Virgil Bradfield from Honolulu; and Dr. Pedro Londono from Columbia.

Dr. (Martin) Kawano became a clinical fellow at Glen Lake in 1952. He survived the atomic bomb blast in Nagasaki, Japan, on August 9, 1945, because he had been at work in a hospital examination room. He came to the United States to study public health at the University of Michigan, but wanted to learn the technique of lung resection, and so he came to Glen Lake.

Although he was one of three Asian doctors, Kawano felt insecure that his dark hair was a disharmony among the blond Scandinavians. He recalled, "When I was sitting with nurses at a table one evening, one of them surprised me. 'The nurses admire your jet-black hair.' . . . My inferiority complex owing to the disagreeable color of my hair in this hospital disappeared completely by her words."

Among Dr. Kawano's patients was Kuwa Yoshida, a Nisei (second-generation Japanese). She helped him navigate the English language and directed him to the Twin City Independent Church, which had services conducted in Japanese by a Nisei minister. Kawano returned to Japan, where he worked as a physician and published a book, *The Cloud and the Light*, about his life experiences.[16]

World War II veterans were still being admitted, even though Glen Lake no longer contracted with the Veterans Administration for care. Manuel Martinez had been infected with TB in Europe during the war. For him, it was a blessing in disguise, because his army unit was transferred to the Pacific Theater, and he stayed behind in a French hospital. In 1953, he had a recurrence of TB as a civilian and was admitted to the sanatorium. He shared a ward with ten other men and received streptomycin, but he didn't need thorax treatment or lung resectioning. After a few months he moved to the East Cottage and was discharged in 1954.[17]

Like Martinez, Howard Johnson was a veteran but did not come directly from the service to the sanatorium. He was working at Flour City Ornamental Iron Works in Minneapolis when he lost weight and began coughing. He took a battery of vocational tests at Glen Lake and, after he was discharged, went to school at Augsburg College. He completed his education at St. Cloud State Teachers' College. "If I hadn't been at the San, I probably would never have gone on to be a teacher," he later said.[18]

The heart hospital in the Children's Building closed in January of 1953. The Variety Heart Club Hospital had opened in Minneapolis and patients were moved there. The Variety Hospital included a forty-bed pediatric unit, with playroom and classroom.

The rate of new tuberculosis infections in the state was slowing. Several factors contributed, including isolation and drug therapy, but a major influence was the intensive testing campaigns that had been conducted by cities and communities across the state. Early detection via skin tests and follow-up X-rays identified active and incipient cases, which meant earlier intervention. With fewer contagious people available to spread disease, there were fewer diagnoses of advanced tuberculosis.

One of Minnesota's most significant contributors to testing was Dr. Kathleen Jordan, whose husband, Dr. Lewis Jordan, was the administrator of the Riverside Sanatorium in Granite Falls. It is estimated that she personally administered more than 2,000,000 skin tests to school children.[19] Dr. Mary Ghostley of Lake Julia Sanatorium at Puposky was also a leader in this campaign in rural Minnesota, as was Dr. Slater at Southwest in Worthington.[20]

Although TB infection was abating in the general population, the state was unable to significantly reduce the death rates for Native Americans and the mentally ill. A 1955 report revealed that two-thirds of the active cases in the mental hospitals developed after admission because state institutions did not require Mantoux tests for all new admissions and employees.

Minnesota Death Rates

Year	Death Rate per 100,000		
	General Population	Native American	Mental Hospital
1936	35.6	385.0	1,083.7
1940	27.3	255.4	858.6
1950	11.1	87.8	309.2
1953	6.9	31.9	180.6

In 1936, the death rate for mental hospital patients was two and a half times as high as for Native Americans. A tuberculosis control program for the two groups, Native Americans and patients in mental hospitals, was started that year, but the results were dramatically different. By 1953, the death rate was six times higher among the mental hospital patients than among Native Americans.

Although there were outreach programs for the Dakota population in southwestern Minnesota, most efforts were concentrated on the reservations near Ah-gwah-ching, the State Sanatorium. Its staff had long worked among the Ojibwe in cooperation with the Minnesota Department of Health. From July 1952 to June 1953, for example, health workers examined or interviewed almost 700 Native American patients from the Leech Lake, Red Lake, and White Earth reservation areas. Diagnostic reports were produced on 3,077 tuberculin tests and 3,797 chest X-rays performed through its outpatient department. In addition, 455 laboratory reports came from the Department of Health.

There was no similar coordinated effort for the mental health patients housed in the state's eight institutions. The 1955 report noted that although the Burns Unit at Anoka had been constructed for a capacity of 250, cottages that were never intended for tuberculosis had been converted and the new capacity was 413. Even so, five percent of mental health patients with TB were still at their home institutions. The Asylum for the Dangerously Insane at St. Peter had a detention unit for twenty patients, and the Minnesota School and Colony at Faribault had a unit for twenty-five tuberculous patients. While Minnesota was among the top states in sanatorium care and TB screening at the local level, it failed miserably at caring for the tuberculous in its institutions.[21]

Nationally, there was success against another contagious disease. Polio, like smallpox, was felled by vaccinations. Because polio is a virus, research focused on protection rather than a cure. Dr. Jonas Salk announced his discovery of a vaccine in 1955, and mass immunizations took place all over the United States. By 1957, the number of new polio cases dropped dramatically, from 58,000 to only 5,600.

By 1955, Glen Lake had served 11,874 patients. Some of those had been admitted multiple times, so the admission total was greater: 15,654. By that year, however, population at the sanatorium dropped so low that the East and West Cottages closed. Tuberculosis mortality per year in Minnesota had gone from 2,042 in 1906 to 128 in less than fifty years. Only 9,589 new cases of TB had been reported to the Minnesota Department of Health from 1950 to 1955, and most of the people were treated as outpatients with chemotherapy. The age of sanatoriums was obviously coming to a close.[22,23]

Several of the smaller county sanatoriums had already transitioned to serving a different population. The aging campuses were costly for the sanatorium districts because of dwindling numbers of patients. Many were operating without a resident medical director because of low salaries and outdated housing. Because sanatoriums were built at a distance from population centers, they had little value to anyone as development property.

In 1951, the commissioners of Todd and Wadena counties sought a legal opinion for clarification of a county nursing home bill passed by the state legislature. They wanted to determine whether the buildings of the jointly owned and operated Fair Oaks Lodge Sanatorium could be converted to a nursing home.

It was an attractive option because in 1950, an amendment to the federal Social Security Act required that payments for medical care be made directly to nursing homes instead of to the person receiving the care. States were also required to license nursing homes in order to participate in the Old Age Assistance program. This meant that the federal government would pay for much of the cost of care, rather than the county or state. It led most of the smaller sanatoriums to consider conversion to what they called old peoples' homes or rest homes.[24]

The Todd/Wadena commissioners' first question for the attorney general was whether the state's initial investment of $50,000 gave it a voice in the disposition of the property. The opinion given by Irving M. Frisch, special assistant to Joseph A.A. Burnquist, was that the buildings were county-owned, but if they were sold the state was entitled to a proportionate reimbursement of the sale.

The next question, "'May such tuberculosis sanatorium building be converted into a nursing home?" received the opinion that a tuberculosis sanatorium established under the provisions of M.S. 376.28 could be discontinued by following the procedure set forth in M.S. 376.54 and then could be converted into a nursing home as provided by Laws 1951, Chapter 610, Section 1, Subdivision 2.[25]

These responses to the Fair Oaks Lodge situation prompted its commissioners and those of Deerwood to close and convert by 1952. Lake Julia and

Oakland Park followed suit in 1954. Buena Vista and Otter Tail converted in 1955. Sand Beach hadn't waited for the attorney general's opinion. It converted to Sunnyside Rest Home on July 1, 1951.

By 1957, it was clear that even a large sanatorium like Glen Lake needed to consider the options. Nopeming Sanatorium was still in operation but had converted one surplus building to a nursing home. An operational review of Glen Lake was conducted by the Citizens League of Minnesota, a non-partisan government policy group. The report pointed out that TB was increasingly a problem of the aged, the poorly paid, and alcoholics, which was resulting in an upward trend of patients unable to pay for their care. The typical patient in the early years had been a young woman. By the late 1950s, a patient was more likely to be a man in his sixties, probably unmarried. The report also stated that the average length of stay had shrunk from over two years to about thirteen months. Glen Lake's discharge rate by death from TB had fallen from over thirty percent annually to less than five percent. The report predicted that specialized hospitals would disappear and be replaced by isolation wards in general hospitals.[26,27]

One suggestion for re-use came from a *Minneapolis Star-Tribune* editorial and echoed Dr. Mariette's opinion of ten years earlier: Why not use the sanitorium as a hospital? The editor said that the same population growth that found Asbury Hospital (later Methodist) moving out to St. Louis Park would demand a hospital further out. "Using Glen Lake Sanatorium as such a hospital is a proposal well worth investigating,"[28] the editorial read.

Two years after the publication of the Citizens' League report, the exact nature of that new use was still being debated. Many beds were empty and the cost of maintenance was a drain on the county's budget. Hennepin County had approached the State of Minnesota more than once, asking it to take over operation of the sanatorium, but it had refused. The need no longer existed for a separate Children's Building at Glen Lake, and it was closed on July 13, 1959.

In 1959, a Hennepin County Sanatorium commissioner, Geri Joseph, initiated a public examiner investigation into accusations of "law violations, favoritism, family 'pull,' waste, and inefficiency" in the operation of Glen Lake tuberculosis sanatorium. The accusations of favoritism and family pull were based on a personnel report she requested. It showed that 100 of the 462 employees were members of families with more than one person on the payroll. An article in the *Minneapolis Morning Tribune*, which had previously employed Joseph as a reporter, detailed several instances of sick leave abuse, absentee employees, and questionable payments made from the payroll and personnel departments. Dr. Frost, Glen Lake superintendent since 1950, resigned from his position shortly thereafter, although he continued as the medical director.[29]

Because the sanatorium was a public institution, a grand jury was seated to investigate the accusations. The grand jury report, issued in June 1959, placed the blame for the irregular practices "squarely on the former three-member sanatorium commission." That commission included Raymond Wright in addition to Geri Joseph, but Dr. Howard Horns had resigned the previous August and a successor had not been named. The report also "took a slap" at the examiner for his "unjustly slanted" report in February. The jury's report did not deny all of the previous report's findings, but it said that "blame for most of the illegal and improper practices must attach to the three sanatorium commissioners." The report noted that almost every practice criticized had been formally approved by the commission.

It also criticized the commission for hiring a private detective to pose as a janitor. Responsibility for having "aided and abetted the sensationalism attendant to the matter" was attributed to the public examiner and two of the commissioners. The report said the jury was also appalled to learn that Dr. Frost had been forced to resign by the commissioners. According to the same newspaper article, Joseph said, "I stand by the public examiner's report and the subsequent actions, most of which were, in my opinion, long overdue."[30]

An editorial published in the *Minneapolis Morning Tribune* in September referred to a "new broom" at Glen Lake, praising a fresh administration and a revised budget that called for a cut of 100 employees.[31]

An entirely new five-member sanatorium commission was soon appointed to govern the sanatorium. The new members were Richard O. Hanson and S. Earl Ainsworth, both county commissioners, and Kenneth Holmquist, Mrs. Walter W. Walker, and Dr. John Edward Twomey. The commissioners installed Owen B. Stubben as administrator and Dr. Victor Funk as the medical director of Glen Lake.[32]

A lengthy letter to the editor from Dorothy Smith criticized the "new broom," citing the increases in director salaries and the additional $20,500 cost of a new administrator. She said he had "all but dispensed with the occupational therapy and rehabilitation programs." As for the cut in employee numbers and a denial of a request for raises, she pointed out that as employees of a contagious disease hospital, it was deceptive to compare their salaries to those in general hospitals. As a sort of last straw in the new broom, she mentioned that employees who patronized the non-profit cafeteria were now also paying for catsup, mustard, and onions for their hamburgers.[33]

The investigation and the grand jury report led to the hiring of a hospital consulting firm to study possible uses for the sanatorium campus. James A. Hamilton and Associates recommended that Glen Lake continue its responsibility for TB care as long as the patient load justified the service. The firm, which was paid $20,000 for its services, came to the same conclusion as 1956 and 1959 recommendations by a Hennepin County Community Chest and Council subcommittee: the sanatorium should become a nursing home.[34] Hamilton and Associates had performed a similar study of Glen Lake in 1950, with the same recommendation.

The newest recommendation, though repetitious, generated some response from the community. The Minnesota Nursing Home Association wanted the sanatorium commission to reject the recommendation of conversion into a county nursing home. The group's president said that "the massive operation proposed for Glen Lake smacks of institutional storage rather than a more homelike atmosphere provided by our smaller private homes." He asserted that private enterprise could build and operate nursing homes more cheaply than converting the sanatorium.

Objections also came from people affiliated with existing nursing homes. Irving Juster's letter to the editor of the *Minneapolis Star* questioned statements about costs and charges and said they were "unfair and misleading."[35] William Goldbert, administrator of Weldwood Nursing Home in Golden Valley, disputed statements about a lack of suitable facilities.[36]

Commissioner Hanson replied that the "Hamilton report was in effect accepted when authorized" six months earlier. "The only question now is implementing its finding," he said.[37]

19

Oak Terrace Nursing Home

T HE PUBLICITY AND DISSENSION seemed to galvanize Hennepin County into once again approaching the state. It succeeded on its third try, in 1961. The state's interest in assuming operation was financial. There were ten state hospitals at the time, and there was overcrowding and an aging population. Of the 10,300 state hospital patients, about 2,000 of them were there only because they were old and had no place to go.[1] When elderly people were in a mental hospital, it was considered psychiatric care and federal funds would not pay for it. By converting the sanatorium to a psycho-geriatric nursing home, the state would be able to collect Medicaid funds instead of using state funding. The state decided to lease the campus from Hennepin County for one dollar per year.[2]

The land for the former Glen Lake Summer Camp had already been sold and was operated as Camp Indian Chief by Arc of Hennepin County as a day camp for people with developmental disabilities. Under the name of Eden Wood Center, it was later operated by True Friends and then by Friendship Ventures for children and adults with mental and physical disabilities.[3,4]

The remainder of the campus was established as Glen Lake State Sanatorium and Oak Terrace Nursing Home in 1961, when legislative action authorized the lease. The law abolished the facility at Walker as the state sanatorium and established the state tuberculosis program at Glen Lake instead. It then established Ah-gwah-ching as the official state nursing home.[5]

On January 22, 1961, the first nursing home patients arrived in a National Guard bus. Glen Lake officially became two institutions, both operated by the state's Department of Public Welfare. There were still two floors of TB

221

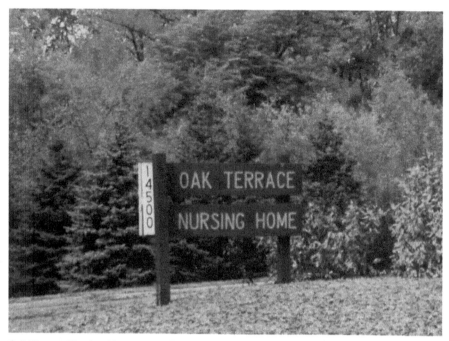

Oak Terrace Nursing Home sign. (Courtesy of Schmidt)

patients, primarily chronic cases who were isolated for active tuberculosis that would probably never become inactive. During 1962, 236 more people would be admitted with a diagnosis of tuberculosis. The average stay was reduced to eight months with the use of chemotherapy.[6]

The remainder of the main building became a geriatric center, essentially a nursing home for elderly patients who needed nursing care beyond that which the state's mental hospitals could provide. The new medical director for both facilities was Dr. Sumner Cohen, who had been at Glen Lake since 1928. Dr. Yue had charge of the tuberculosis service. Melvin Dray replaced Stubben as the administrator.[7] Maury Treberg was hired as the business manager in 1962, and then succeeded Dray when he retired. In later years, Dr. Aurel Sulciner, a native of Romania and a Holocaust survivor, served as the medical director.

The sanatorium employees were invited to continue employment at the facility, but had to pass the state's civil service exam to do so. Those who stayed composed about half of the workforce.

Judy Scholer was one of the new hires. When she came to work at Oak Terrace Nursing Home, she expected to be a hospital aide in the nursing home. She was assigned to one of the tuberculosis floors instead because she had a positive Mantoux.[8]

Some of the new employees, like Margaret Anderson, were returning to familiar territory. She had worked in the Children's Building from 1948 until 1951. Anderson came back to work in 1967, after staying home to raise a family. She felt there was still some of the sanatorium aura on Main East, where she was a nurse on a rehabilitation ward. By her retirement in 1986, though, much about healthcare had changed and it seemed to her to have become an industry. One change she disliked was absence of the white nursing uniform, complete with a cap that identified the school nurses graduated from. The nursing home dress code was more casual, to convey a more homey atmosphere. Anderson wore her full nursing uniform to her retirement party.[9]

Charlotte Crowe also worked a split shift, so to speak. She joined the sanatorium staff in 1949, became the assistant nursing director, and left in 1961. After returning to college for two years, she came back to be director of nurses and stayed for ten years. For her, there wasn't much difference in the daily operation, just fewer patients and different physical issues.[10]

Betty Carroll saw the changes from a different viewpoint. When she worked as a social worker in the sanatorium, the average age of patients was about thirty. And although people stayed two or three years and she got to know them well, they anticipated a return home. When she returned to work in the nursing home in 1966, the residents were much older and most had been institutionalized for decades. People would ask her, "How can you stand it?" But the atmosphere was not depressive for her. Most of the residents were appreciative, and some were affectionate. During the sanatorium years, she lived on campus, and it had seemed like a family. At the nursing home, it was just a daytime situation. Still, she found the nursing home more rewarding, because she had found it harder to establish a relationship with the 350 sanatorium patients she was assigned to help.[11]

A unique feature of the environment in the blended facility was the stability of the medical and support staff. There was a tradition of care inherited from the sanatorium. That care included the social services involvement dating from the 1920s.

Paulette Anderson, Oak Terrace social worker, expressed her opinion that the "strong sense of history with regards to the quality of care has really been a benefit to the nursing home. It would be rather uncommon to find a nursing home that has the kind of background that this facility does." On the other hand, she said, the historical legacy could be frustrating at times. People did things a certain way for thirty-five years and wanted to continue doing so into the future.[12]

The recreation department was another unique feature. A small group of residents went swimming at Courage Center twice a week. Another group bowled regularly in Hopkins, complete with bowling banquet at Bursch's Cafe. Volunteers brought in pets before that was an accepted part of therapy. Teenagers serving sentences for juvenile court were encouraged to come and fraternize with patients. Raised garden beds allowed residents in wheelchairs to exercise their green thumbs. For a while there were even some chickens in residence, too. Staff from all departments would provide entertainment, including gurney races during an annual summer picnic and winter talent shows in the auditorium.[13]

The family feeling of the sanatorium, with ex-patients staying on as employees, and family members working in various capacities, was carried on by people such as the Haugers. Jarvis Hauger, Oak Terrace business manager for fourteen and a half years, recalled the camaraderie with other employees. They formed a bowling team and produced plays for the patients. Both of his parents had worked at Glen Lake—his father, Jacob, for forty-two years and his mother, Ruth, as a teacher in the Children's Building for thirty-six years.[14]

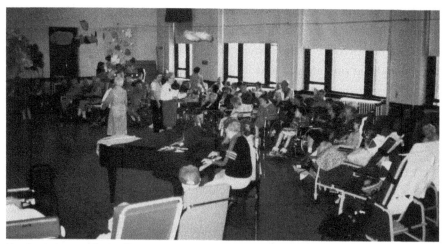

Nursing home residents. (Courtesy of the Minnesota Historical Society)

Dora Cohen, dietician at both institutions, remembered the real feeling of community. "Employees would work overtime for any special event or party. No one expected to be paid for that. It was just part of good will."[15]

Ramona Ebert-Pockrandt recalled the home environment that she experienced as a child when her mother healed in the sanatorium. Ramona felt it was still there when she herself became an Oak Terrace employee.[16]

Norma Anderson, volunteer coordinator at Oak Terrace, noticed that employees during the nursing home days developed the same kind of feeling. Prospective volunteers echoed that impression. Some actually "shopped" nursing homes to find one in which to do volunteer work. Norma said that when people came into the place and saw the tender loving care that was being given to the people, they would decide it was the place for them to volunteer. At one point, there were 1,000 volunteers on the rolls. Anderson told her children, "When my time comes and I have to go to a nursing home, I want to go to Oak Terrace."[17]

There was a deliberate decision to call the new nursing home arrivals residents instead of patients. Maury Treberg was quick to remind employees that, "This is their home; we just work here." The first group of new residents came from St. Peter State Hospital, the largest of the state's mental institutions and "usually regarded as the most rickety." The next transfer included the tuberculous patients from Ah-gwah-ching.[18]

In addition to St. Peter, people came from Anoka, Cambridge, Brainerd, Faribault, Fergus Falls, Moose Lake, and Willmar. The residents from the state hospitals had complex medical and behavioral disabilities that did not allow them to live successfully in a community nursing home.

New patients were occasionally admitted to the tuberculosis floors. One of them was Raymond Sotelo. His tuberculosis was most likely job-related, and he was admitted to the TB floor of the nursing home in 1969. Sotelo could walk around on that floor and through the tunnels, but couldn't be on the floors where the nursing home residents lived. When he was discharged and could work only part-time, his employer initially told him they didn't have a position for him. They relented, and he worked half days while he built up his strength. Coincidentally, he married Gloria Yberra, who had spent her childhood in the Children's Building.[19]

The Oak Terrace post office was discontinued, and mail was processed through the Glen Lake branch of the Minnetonka post office. The new address was 14500 County Road 62, with a ZIP code of 55345.[20]

Terrace Topics was revived in newsletter format as *Terrace Topics II*. The Department of Public Welfare continued to offer a library for the residents, and its own medical library was relocated to available space in the main building.

To accommodate the needs of nursing home residents versus tuberculosis patients, some remodeling was needed. Elevator controls were lowered so people in wheelchairs could reach them. There were no elevator operators as there were in the sanatorium. Bathroom doors were made wider, wash basins lowered, and handrails installed. Wheelchair ramps were created so residents could go outdoors, and a lift was installed in the nursing home van.

The seventy-five-acre campus and large buildings provided the residents with a fair amount of freedom balanced with the protection they needed. The nursing care and rehabilitation services gave them a special quality of life that many of them had not been able to have in the traditional state hospital setting.[21] Although the clientele had changed, the focus on entertainment and occupational therapy for the people living in the building had not. Community organizations and church groups helped to celebrate holidays.

The nursing home later began to serve adults of any age with medical or behavioral issues that couldn't be provided in a community setting. The care of people permanently and severely injured in accidents became a specialty, and they lived on the old "sun" floor, Fifth Main.[22]

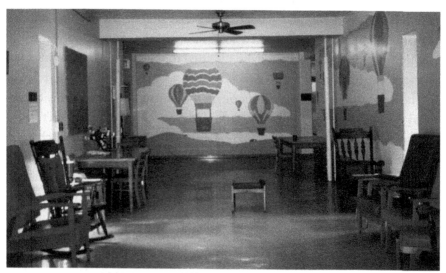

Balloon mural. (Courtesy of Barker)

By 1967, the patient census for tuberculosis was down to fifty-one. The sanatorium was still accredited by the Joint Commission on Hospital Accreditation and continued to work with the U.S. Public Health Service in the testing of new drugs.[23] It also participated, along with Ah-gwah-ching, in a Minnesota Nursing Home Study sponsored by the National Institute of Mental Health. For a short while, the campus hosted a Treatment Center for Emotionally Disturbed Children until it was moved to a permanent location at Lino Lakes.

The last tuberculosis patient was discharged on paper and admitted to Oak Terrace Nursing home in 1976. Glen Lake wasn't officially closed until 1980, when Minnesota Statute 357 removed Glen Lake State Sanatorium as a state institution.

The Department of Public Welfare was renamed the Department of Human Services. More patients arrived when two state hospitals closed completely—Hastings in 1978 and Rochester in 1982.

In 1977, the superintendent's residence in the north part of the campus was leased to West Suburban Alano Society for use as a counseling center for alcoholics and their families. Also in that year, the nurses' residence was leased to Nexus, a rehabilitative program for released felons.

Part of the Children's Building was given over to Happy Hearts Daycare. The child care facility was the brainchild of an affirmative-action committee. Members were charged with enhancing the quality of work life in general and recommended an on-site day care. A community survey revealed a demand, and it opened in the mid-1980s as the first day-care facility on a state campus.[24]

The drunk tank in the east wing, used in the TB days for drying out alcoholics and subduing boisterous patients, was transformed into a Christian chapel. The stained glass window, with the Psalm Twenty-three theme of the good shepherd, was designed by the daughter of a chaplain. Funding came from organizations in the community and parishes. In addition to providing a non-denominational place to worship or meditate, it also carried the symbolism of change.

Various state chaplains came out to conduct services until a full-time chaplain, Neil Hering, was hired. He was impressed by the campus.

I remember thinking, "this is a nursing home? This is just one nursing home?" One of the special things about it being so big is that the people love to roam, both inside and the grounds that are beautiful and it gives them an outlet. And the auditorium. I mean, what community nursing home has a huge place that we can use for therapeutic recreation and worship?[25]

The state rabbi, Rabbi Barry Wolf, began regular visits to Jewish residents and a room was remodeled, painted blue, and designated for their use.[26]

By the mid-1980s, the building was showing its age. The floors of the stairwell landings had small depressions in the terrazzo, showing where thousands of feet had pivoted on their way to the next flight of stairs. Except for window air conditioners in strategic areas, the buildings were not air conditioned. New technologies that needed special wiring, such as computers, were difficult to accommodate in a building with walls of concrete and brick.

Not all parts of the building were inadequate. The boiler inspector told Don Jones, maintenance engineer, that "the boilers would probably last another 100 years." The metal parts and bricks had some work done on them, but the boilers were essentially those put in place in when the power plant was built. Two of the pumps were original and still used on a daily basis.[27]

It was hard to keep the building in compliance with all of the regulations, however. The Health Department came every year to do an audit. There were federal Medicaid and Medicare regulations to follow, as well as fire marshal inspections to be ready for. The cost for installing fire-suppression sprinklers was $400,000 in 1980. Not only did the regulations seem to change every year, but one group's regulations sometimes conflicted with another's.

The competition for funding was keen at the Capitol, and legislators were more generous funding remodeling for the state hospitals they owned, rather than for a campus they leased. In 1989, the state legislature responded to a request from the Department of Human Services and approved the closure of Oak Terrace Nursing Home.

To celebrate seventy-five years of combined medical service to Hennepin County and the State of Minnesota, a homecoming was held at Oak Terrace Nursing Home on August 19, 1990. Former patients and employees enjoyed visiting and looking through old photographs and other memorabilia. The Community Relations Department hosted a volunteer recognition party and conducted tours. The Minnetonka Friends of the Library sponsored a presentation by Frederick Manfred, during which he read from his sanatorium-based book, *Boy Almighty*. Norma Anderson compiled and published a booklet of interviews titled *San Memories*.

With help from Paragon Cable's Hopkins Studio and producer Steve Perkins, the event was videotaped and became part of a local cable-access documentary. Also included were previously taped interviews of former staff and patients by Colleen Spadaccini, Doris Solie, Marge Kozachok, and Mary Krugerud. The documentary, titled *From Beginning to End*, was broadcast on local cable access channels. Later that year, the documentary won a local Cable Ace award in the Minnesota History division.

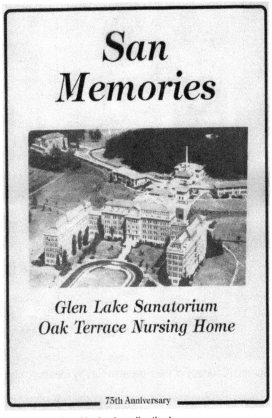

San
Memories

Glen Lake Sanatorium
Oak Terrace Nursing Home

75th Anniversary

San Memories. (Author's collection)

Several employees contributed squares to quilts that represented Glen Lake and Oak Terrace. Margaret Kienzle got the idea for her square on a quilt from the TB patients who applauded a performance in the auditorium. She remembered the patients clapping as they were

> . . . lying on the litter, flat, watching the performance, and it just hit me as I stood in the door of the dining room as the performance was going on. It just stayed in my memory. What a beautiful thing! They can't even get up. They had to be flat on their backs and yet they could show their appreciation with the hands all coming up. It was very inspiring.[29]

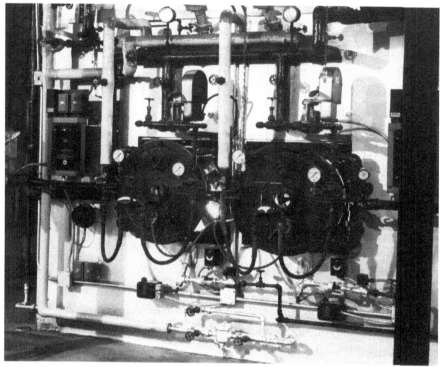

Boilers. (Courtesy of the Hennepin History Museum)

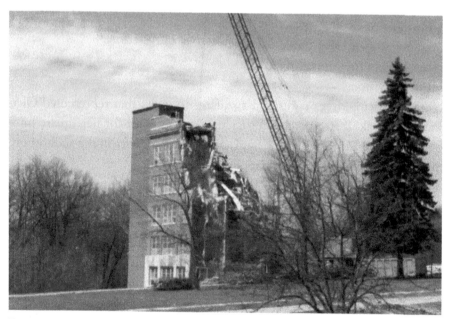

Demolition. (Courtesy of Schmidt)

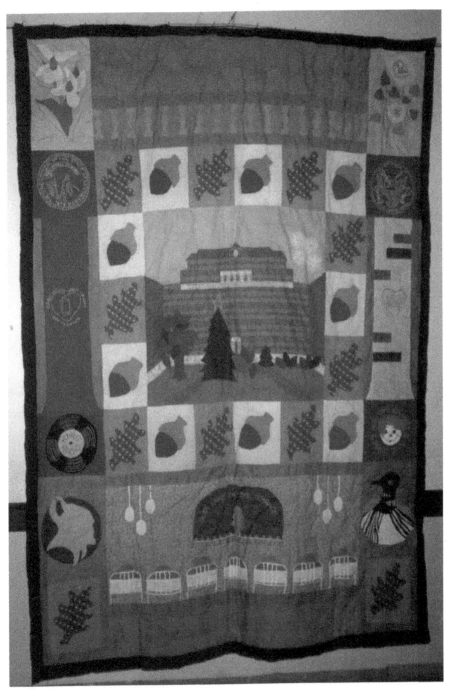

Glen Lake Sanitorium quilt. (Author's collection)

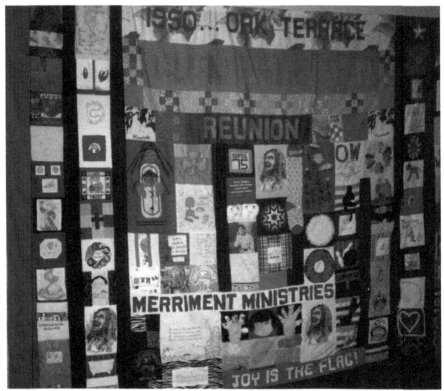

Reunion quilt. (Author's collection))

Many people mourned the closing. Myrtle Murk echoed Norma Anderson when she said, "I am really sad it is closing down. I felt that when I became the age when I had to be put into an institution like this, this is where I'd want to come. I'm really sad. Really. It's an era that's going to be gone forever."[30]

In 1991, the nursing home closed. Together the two institutions had cared for more than 17,000 people. The property transferred back to Hennepin County and the buildings were demolished in 1993. It did not go easy. Someone underestimated the sturdiness of the structures, and many people gathered to watch the wrecking ball bounce off the walls.

"Although the county was advised in 1991 that the facility was eligible for listing on the National Register of Historic Places, it is doubtful whether this information was seriously considered." The site was documented to the standards of the Historic American Building Survey (HABS) and made available on the Library of Congress's Prints and Photographs Online Catalog.

The Preservation Alliance of Minnesota said in its newsletter, "It is believed that Hennepin County would like to develop the seventy-five-acre site as a golf course, which seems an ironic end for the facility just as tuberculosis is making a comeback in the United States."[31]

The land did become a golf course, the Glen Lake Golf and Practice Center operated by the Three Rivers Park District. Its nine-hole course encompasses the original campus in Minnetonka and part of the former children's camp in Eden Prairie.

The Glen Lake Children's Camp was placed on the National Register of Historic Places in 1999. The Eden Prairie, Minnesota, City Council named the Glen Lake Children's Camp a Heritage Preservation site on April 16, 2013. A stone monument placed to honor Mr. and Mrs. George H. Christian for their efforts in establishing the Glen Lake Children's Camp remains on the grounds. The dining hall, a dormitory, and a garage date back to the camp's years of operation, and it might be one of only two tuberculosis children's camp sites still existing in the United States.

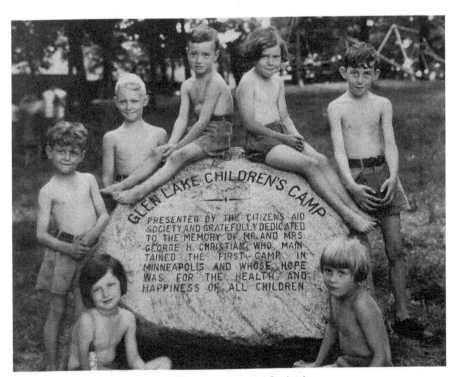

Dedication rock. (Courtesy of the Minnesota Historical Society)

20

Measuring Success

WERE SANATORIUMS SUCCESSFUL? It depends whom you ask and how you measure success.

If you were to ask Irwin W. Sherman, who wrote *Twelve Diseases That Changed the World*, he would probably say, "No." In his book he points to the sanatoriums' "lack of success in curing the disease."[1] If you define "cure" as direct responsibility for eradication or as 100-percent recovery rates, then he is right, they weren't successful.

Dr. J. Arthur Myers and medical historian Leonard Wilson saw success in the larger picture: a collaborative tuberculosis control system. The Minnesota State Medical Association's Public Health Committee, formed in 1924, had members from every organization that was active in tuberculosis work. The committee helped initiate and promote projects and attempted to keep any one program or organization from dominating state and local efforts. Minnesota gained national attention for this clearing-house approach to eradication. A Medical Association report from 1962 noted that the Minnesota Method of Tuberculosis Control was still attracting attention from all over the world. The method can be summarized as local control with state organizational oversight. The sanatoriums, with intake services and outpatient clinics, were very much a part of that method.[2]

Dr. Ejvind Fenger, a specialist in bone and joint tuberculosis at Glen Lake, would probably have said that success depends on the type of tuberculosis. Before the 1940s, the greatest improvement was for people infected with tuberculosis of the bone. In 1927, the average length of stay for someone with bone TB was about 1,200 days. That average was halved by 1938. Heliotherapy was the only treatment prior to chemotherapy that produced dramatic results on a specific type of tuberculosis.[3]

Leslie Maitland, an architectural historian, defined a different type of success in her article about the design of tuberculosis hospitals. She provides evidence that lessons learned in the building of tuberculosis sanatoriums influenced the construction of homes and "form a foundation of the architecture with which we live today." As the construction of the sanatoriums evolved, housing design changed as well. Houses of the early twentieth century began to feature more windows, open porches, and better ventilation systems. Easy-to-clean building materials, such as tile and linoleum, replaced carpeting. Washable fabrics replaced heavy wools and drapery. Design changes reflected an increased awareness of the need for light, air, and a clean living environment.[4]

Dr. Henry Bracken, executive secretary of the State Board of Health, in effect said "yes" to the question of sanatoria's success through his strong support of state aid for construction and maintenance of public sanatoriums. Bracken said that dedicated housing is a beneficial, protective measure for the entire community. He pointed out that the sanatorium was not merely for the treatment of an individual. Whenever the cost was discussed, it was usually because taxpayers or legislators asked why state aid was available for tuberculosis and not for other hospitalized diseases. Bracken justified funding for tuberculosis on the same greater-good principle as state aid for public school education. By isolating those who were infectious, sanatoriums may have saved thousands of lives.[5]

Presenting hard data on the success of a sanatorium cure is nearly impossible. During the peak years of their operation, very few, if any, sanatoriums tracked discharged patients or did comparison evaluations or controlled experiments. The death rate was commonly used as the measure of sanatorium success.

The accompanying chart shows a sharp drop in the actual number of deaths in Minnesota due to tuberculosis starting in 1918. By that time, there were nineteen sanatoriums and tuberculosis wards operating in the state. From 1907 until 1918, about 1,000 people with active tuberculosis had been removed from homes and workplaces and admitted to sanatoriums. That, combined with education and sanitation campaigns, probably helped to slow the spread of the disease.[6]

However, early reporting in Minnesota omitted anyone who came in and died within thirty days, because the sanatorium commission believed the patients were too far gone to have received any benefit from the sanatorium, anyway.

Although summary reports are available for most of the county sanatoriums, the original patient records and admissions books are not. Therefore, the consistency of recorded thirty-day admissions among the institutions is unknown. Also unknown is the accuracy of duplicated admissions (returning patients counted as new).

In the accompanying table, sanatorium admissions marked with an asterisk indicate that the number may reflect duplicated admissions, thereby lowering the morbidity percentage. The statistics end with the year 1947, when streptomycin was available in limited amounts at Glen Lake and Mineral Springs and possibly not at all at the other sanatoriums.

Minnesota Sanatorium Death Rates Ending 1947

Name	Unduplicated Admissions	Deaths	Deaths as Percentage
Buena Vista	782	170	22%
Deerwood	699	135	19%
Fair Oaks Lodge	868	202	23%
Glen Lake	9,587	3,011	31%
Lake Julia	1,337	341	25%
Mineral Springs	1,801	495	27%
Minnesota State	10,833*	1,660	15%
Nopeming	5,645	710	12%
Oakland Park	880	300	34%
Otter Tail	1,147	364	32%
Ramsey/Ancker	7,880*	2,535	29%
Riverside	1,091	327	30%
Sand Beach	946	329	35%
Southwestern	1,454	272	19%
Sunnyrest	1,471	413	28%
Totals	**46,421**	**11,264**	**24%**

Source: Myers, *Invited and Conquered*

Some of the variations can be explained. Glen Lake and Ramsey/Ancker accepted advanced cases. Mineral Springs also accepted some advanced cases because of its consultant physician relationship with Mayo Clinic. Some sanatoriums took only patients with incipient tuberculosis who recovered

Buena Vista Sanatorium,
Wabasha, Minn,

SUMMARY FOR YEAR ENDING December 31, 1921

Classified According to					I. All Patients who Stayed over 30 Days										II. Time of Resid				
LESION	SYMPTOMS A	B	C	Turban	Sputum	Cases	App. Cure	Arrest-ed	App. Arr.	Quies-cent	Impr.	Prog.	Died	Av'rage Resi-dence Weeks	CLASS	Cases	15 Days or Less	15 to 30 Days	1 Month to 3 Months
Incipient	2 1	1		I	O				2	1			42	Incipient	5		1	
				I	†	3 1			1					Moderately Advanced				
				‡										Far Advanced	5	1		
Moderately Advanced	1 1	1		I	O'										14	4	2	2
				I	†													
				II	O	1			1	1	1	1	22	TOTAL	24	5	3	2
				II	†	3												
				III	O													
				III	†									III. Conditions of Sputum (Posit:			
Far Advanced	1 4	3		I	O									CLASS	Cases	Apparently Cured	
				II	†	8			2	6				Incipient	5	Pos. / Neg.	
				III	O						19			Moderately Advanced	5	Pos. / Neg.	
				III	†				2	6				Far Advanced	14	Pos. / Neg.	
TOTAL	4 7	5				4			4	17				TOTAL	24	Pos. / Neg.	

NOTE—* = No sputum report available. † = No turban classification. Cases not reported, owing to lack of information. 1 died after 9 days res. 1 14 15

Buena Vista Sanatorium records. (Courtesy of the Minnesota Historical Society)

quickly. At some sanatoriums, people on the verge of dying were transferred to a hospital, and their deaths do not appear in the sanatorium record. A few of the smaller sanatoriums lacked a house physician or had continued turnover in medical staff, which affected the quality of care. However, measured against the conventional wisdom that gave people with active tuberculosis a fifty-fifty chance of dying, sanatoriums were generally considered to increase chances of survival.

It is also difficult to determine whether the financial investment in sanatoriums was worth the final result. Up until about 1950, the cost of operating a sanatorium was rarely questioned. There was no cure, and fatality rates remained high enough to make long-term hospitalization an acceptable option.

An increase in expenditures in the late 1940s triggered questions about the cost of care. Possibly the greatest contributor was the transformation of tuberculosis treatment from passive rest and food to surgery and chemotherapy. Surgery could decrease a length of stay, but the cost was not balanced by savings realized by fewer days of care.

Many pulmonary resections were performed at Glen Lake on patients with moderately advanced to advanced tuberculosis. Dr. Martin Kawano studied the results of resections performed at Glen Lake from the years 1928 to 1948 and found that nine resection surgeries were performed. Three patients died within six months. Of the remaining six, only one had died by July 1953. After antibiotics came into common use, the occurrence of surgeries rose from five in 1949 (all still alive four years later) to 168 in 1952. Of a total 318 surgeries from 1949 to 1953, eight patients died within six months of the operation, and only one other died by 1953.[7]

Without additional data from other studies nationwide, no judgment can be made about the overall effectiveness of lung surgery. At Glen Lake, the post-surgery death rate was 2.3 percent over the period of the study. It stands in comparison to the sanatorium's percentage of discharges by death, which was 23.7 percent in 1948. Patients would have been aware of what looked to them like success, and evidently they acted accordingly and opted for lung surgery.

Tuberculosis did seem to be in retreat. The incidence of new cases had dropped only from 100 per 100,000 of population in 1930 to eighty per 100,000 in 1950, but the U.S. death rate for the same period went from seventy per 100,000 down to twenty. Whether that can be attributed to any one effort is debatable.

Sanatoriums provided other benefits not quantifiable in determining success. For families where tuberculosis was present, sanatoriums relieved them of the risk of living with a contagious person. At-home caregivers were exposed to bacteria when they lacked proper equipment to handle contaminated materials.

In 1913, the University of Minnesota published a research paper by Herbert G. Lampson. His "Study on the Spread of Tuberculosis in Families" reported on examinations of forty tuberculous families and fifteen families that had no tuberculosis. In the tuberculous families, 207 individuals were examined and 138 individuals showed evidence of tuberculous infection, or 66.3 percent. In ten of those families, every person examined was infected. In the fifteen non-tuberculous families, eighty individuals were examined. Only two showed evidence of infection and two were suspected.[8]

The Botten family of Montevideo is one of many in which multiple members contracted tuberculosis. Two sisters died at home, and their brother entered Riverside Sanatorium. After Ruby and her nephew Larry died at Glen Lake, no other family members developed active tuberculosis.[9]

Sanatoriums also relieved family members of nursing a long-term invalid at home. Also, patients who tried to take the cure at home found that the regimen of fresh air, rest, and good food could be difficult to follow in a household of active people. Some patients who left against medical advice returned to the sanatorium to complete their program.

A sanatorium also taught and encouraged a healthful lifestyle that many continued after discharge. Norma Anderson recalled that Ruby Hegg, a former TB patient, once scolded her for trying to pick up something from the floor. Hegg fetched a paper towel to retrieve the item and put it in the wastebasket. She explained that a floor is contaminated and shouldn't be touched.[10]

Despite the lack of proven successes, Glen Lake Sanatorium garnered praise and recognition for its administration and innovations. Glen Lake was the largest sanatorium in Minnesota and one of the largest in the United States. Others of comparable size were the Arkansas Tuberculosis Sanatorium (state-run), Olive View Sanatorium in Los Angeles (county), Chicago Municipal Sanatorium (city), William H. Maybury Sanatorium in Detroit (city-county), Sea View Hospital in New York (city), Pennsylvania Sanatorium in South Mountain (state), and Firland Sanatorium in Seattle (city). In terms of research and reputation, the best were considered to be Jewish National Sanatorium in Denver and the Trudeau Sanatorium at Saranac Lake, New York.

Glen Lake was in the vanguard of sanatoriums adopting administrative innovations. It was one of the first to have a Medical Records Department that maintained and organized patient records for research purposes as well as ongoing care. Other uses for that information ranged from small presentations and published papers to national symposiums. Glen Lake's physicians and department heads regularly shared what they learned. In 1937, they held forty-seven internal medical and clinical pathology meetings; published thirty-one articles in national medical journals; gave seventy-nine lectures to nurses, nursing students, and medical students; and made fifty-two presentations to external organizations.[11]

Glen Lake was able to successfully implement what would one day be called a "continuous improvement model" because the medical staff was stable and loyal. Six physicians spent more than twenty years each on staff: Ernest Mariette, Sumner Cohen, Ejvind Fenger, Victor Funk, Leonard Larson, and Peter Mattill. They set high standards and met them, exceeding their own goal of hospital accreditation by becoming the first sanatorium in the nation to do so. The Medical Staff Meeting Minutes reveal a group of physicians who, under the guidance of a visionary director, strove to provide a cheerful and optimistic atmosphere for people who had an incurable, infectious disease and encountered death daily.

Under Dr. Mariette's direction, Glen Lake embraced the concept of holistic medicine even before the word "holism" was coined in 1926. Mariette's belief that the contented patient is a healing patient resulted in the sanatorium's liberal visiting hours, flavorful meals, and a variety of entertainments. One of the aspects of sanatorium life that is difficult for a modern person to understand, though, is the willingness of people to stay in bed for years. Psychological and sociological studies offer theories about institutionalization, the subjugation to ritual, and the childlike acceptance of rules.

It's important, then, to realize how few options were available to anyone stricken with tuberculosis prior to 1950. It was a capricious disease. Some family members would sicken; others wouldn't. A patient who seemed to be on the road to recovery would hemorrhage and die. Patients who were expected to die would rally from the brink and live. It was, and still is, a disease that carries a stigma. Chapter thirty of a medical book from 1939 is titled, "Tuberculosis, Syphilis, and Gonorrhea." In 2016, within the national Center for Disease Control, tuberculosis statistics were published under the umbrella heading of HIV/AIDS, Viral Hepatitis, STD (sexually transmitted disease), and TB prevention.[12]

For a substantial portion of the sanatorium population in the early twentieth century, hospitalization provided a considerable improvement in living conditions. Some patients at the sanatorium lived in near luxury compared to their families, especially during the Great Depression. Oil- or wood-burning stoves were the norm for many dwellings, while the sanatorium had central heating. The Harmsen family and others from Minneapolis lived in cold-water flats—so-called because the apartments had no running hot water. There was a steady supply of it at Glen Lake. Some homes did not have indoor plumbing and relied on backyard outhouses. Juanita Seck, whose first job was at Glen Lake in 1939, came from a home in Robbinsdale that didn't have running water. She thought her apartment in the ground level of the West Wing was ". . . high-class living, bathtub, indoor toilets, and all that."[13]

The Rural Electrification Act, authorized by Congress in 1936, took some time to enact, so kerosene lanterns still illuminated most farms, with intermittent electricity supplied via windmills and storage batteries. Glen Lake generated its own power in the early years, ensuring consistent delivery of electricity for lights, refrigeration, and fans.

Obviously, living in a sanatorium could be terrifying, depressing, dull, and confining. One man refused to be interviewed about his sanatorium stay almost forty years later, saying that the experience was so painful that he preferred not to relive it. Some former patients had mixed feelings about their sanatorium life. In a letter to Dr. Cohen, Frederick Manfred said, "This is a hell-hole, though it is a wonderful place, too."[14,15]

The pain and repercussions of separation from family could be unimaginable. When Frances Lange became a widow in 2006, she told people she felt that she had already had her widowhood, in her first year of marriage. Her husband, Gil, entered Glen Lake just before their first wedding anniversary. Frances herself became a patient a few months later. They couldn't see each other often, because Gil was on strict bed for a year and a half. When Gil felt discouraged and didn't want to live, Dr. Mattill asked her what she thought could be done. Frances said, "I think it would help if you gave us a leave." He did, and the weekend together away from the sanatorium improved Gil's attitude.[16]

For Gloria Yberra Sotelo, who had entered Glen Lake as an infant, it was the only home she knew. Her return to her real home at age twelve was terrifying. Her parents were immigrants from Mexico and spoke primarily Spanish in their apartment home on Tenth Avenue South in Minneapolis. Gloria had been raised speaking only English. She knew she had a family but rarely saw them because of the expense of traveling out to Glen Lake. There was no bond with them. At home, everything from food to bathing facilities was so different from what she was accustomed to. Gloria was shocked that she had to share a bed with her sister in a small apartment that was heated by only an oil burner. It was so overwhelming that she would cry sometimes, "I want to go home." And her dad would say, "You are already home."

For a whole year Gloria prayed that she would get sick and go back out to the sanitorium, and perhaps her prayers were answered. She developed pneumonia, and her mother took her to General Hospital. When they found out she had had tuberculosis at one time, they transferred her to Glen Lake. Gloria lived at the Children's Building for another two years, and the next time she was ready for discharge, social workers recommended that she not go back home. Gloria became a ward of the state and was taken in by a family whose daughter was a heart patient. As an adult she wondered why she wasn't more exposed to the outside world so she would have been prepared.[17]

After his discharge, Don Rivers wrote an open letter to Glen Lake patients and published it in *Terrace Topics*:

> I'd lie there, after the lights had gone out, with the feeling that the head of my bed consisted of prison bars that separated me from all the glamour of the world outside. And I'd start getting a little bitter, wondering if existence were worth it, worth the months and months of inactivity, the monotony of a hospital routine, the peas-in-a-pod sameness of days. Now, thinking back on all the moonlit nights I've enjoyed since then, I realize the price was little enough.[18]

LuDean Harmsen Pontius, who lived in the Children's Building for most of her childhood, doesn't tell a lot of people about her time at the sanatorium, but when she does mention it, people say, "You poor thing." She replies, "Don't feel sorry for me. I had a better life than a lot of kids. I was so spoiled."[19]

Phyllis Burns, who came to the sanitorium as a cadet nurse during World War II, summarized her feelings as an employee, saying, "It was a marvelous community of caring. Never have I seen the equal to the nursing and medical care that was given at Glen Lake. I've always been proud of having been a part of that."[20]

In a 1990 interview, Dr. Funk reflected on the sanatorium's atmosphere: "I think it was surprising that this was an optimistic and cheerful place to work."[21]

After a cure for tuberculosis was discovered, the need to provide a special place for recovery diminished. "We worked ourselves out of job," said Dr. Tsai.[22]

Chemotherapy was the primary reason for the decline of tuberculosis in the U.S., but socioeconomic changes had led to an improved standard of living for many people, which decreased their chances of being infected. Educating the general populace about infections also contributed to a decline. And, like many contagious diseases, tuberculosis seems to follow an epidemic curve, although a very long one. Perhaps the sanatoriums merely helped to hasten the inevitable end of its life cycle.[23]

After chemotherapy came into common use, the cost-benefit questions became more common. Costs were, in fact, rising dramatically. Glen Lake's cost of operation rose from $758,420 in 1930 to $2,157,016 in 1950. The per-diem price of care went from $2.74 to $9.59 during the same time period. Annual inflation was 1.59 percent over those two decades, accounting for less than two dollars of the per diem increase.[24]

The total cost of operation for Glen Lake from 1916 to January 1948 was $23,118,722. With total patient admissions at 12,323 (duplicated), the cost per patient per admission was $1,876. Although that figure was not adjusted for inflation over the thirty-two years of operation, it would equal about $18,000 in 2016.

Most people with tuberculosis are now cured by following a strict six-month drug regimen. Costs to treat a non-multi-drug resistant tuberculosis patient in the early 2000s were estimated at $17,000, about the same as a lengthy sanatorium cure.

In 1960, Dr. Mervyn M. Williams, from Ah-gwah-ching Sanatorium, addressed the Minnesota Legislature and said, "We lifted the fear—nobody's afraid of tuberculosis anymore. But never will we out-treat and extinguish tuberculosis. We have improved our position, but the enemy is still there."[25]

In 1961, an article in *Minnesota's Health* stressed, "If tuberculosis is to be eradicated it must be done before the bacillus produces so many drug-resistant mutants that drug therapy is no longer effective."[26]

The improper use of antibiotics, including patients who quit taking the medication before a cure, has indeed led to multidrug-resistant tuberculosis (MDR). Drug resistant forms can be caused by non-compliant patients not completing the full course of antibiotics. The cost of treating a patient with an extreme form of MDR can soar to nearly half a million dollars.[27]

Directly observed therapy, known as DOT, is one approach to preventing MDR. A person with tuberculosis takes the medicine in a clinic, home, or other structured setting under the observation of a health care worker to ensure that the course of treatment is completed and a cure is achieved.[28]

Worldwide, tuberculosis ranks alongside HIV/AIDS as the leading cause of death from a contagious disease. In 2015, an estimated 1.8 million people died from it. Tuberculosis is an opportunistic disease, so people with existing health issues, such as HIV, are more at risk of developing active tuberculosis than someone in good health. Of the people who died from TB in 2015, 400,000 of them were co-infected with HIV.[29]

Tuberculosis is still with us in Minnesota, too. The state's tuberculosis rate in 2015 was 2.7 cases per 100,000 persons. There were 150 cases of active tuberculosis reported that year, most of them occurring in Hennepin and Ramsey counties. Two of the TB cases reported in 2015 died.[30]

Minnesota's rate is nearly the same as that of the United States, which saw 3.0 cases per 100,000 persons in 2015. Of the 9,557 cases of tuberculosis reported in that year, tuberculosis among foreign-born persons accounted for sixty-six percent.[31]

In spite of MDR tuberculosis, the era of large institutions dedicated solely to the isolation and care of people with tuberculosis is unlikely to return. Hospitalization for a half year or more is a solution too extreme for a modern population to consider.

Appendix A
Glen Lake Sanatorium and
Oak Terrace Nursing Home Personnel

Listed below are just a few of the physicians, nurses, and support staff who worked at the sanatorium and/or the nursing home, some for more than thirty years.

Name	Occupation/Years Employed/Notes
Ainsworth, S. Earl	Sanatorium commission member, 1960, county commissioner.
Allen, Leona	Maid, 38+ years.
Akerson, Walter	Carpenter, 43 years, 1923–1966.
Anderson, Axel	Utility man, 34 years.
Baldwin, Frederick	Physician, about 1918–1920.
Baxter, Beulah	1946 (cadet nurse) to 1985 (nurse at Oak Terrace).
Bell, John W.	Sanatorium commission, 1913–1919, University of Minnesota faculty.
Bendes, J. Harry	Physician and heliotherapy specialist, 1921–1927, went to Rockford (Illinois) Municipal Sanatorium, then private practice.
Bendis, John	Elevator operator, 29 years, former patient.
Bentilla, Edith	Nurse, 31 years.
Bergren, Lillian	Occupational therapy, 33 years.
Bergren, Olaf	Lab technician, 30 years.
Biship, Marjorie	Outpatient clinic, 34 years.
Boquist, Harold S.	Physician in residency in 1921, staff member in outpatient clinic, died in 1934 of strep infection.
Borak, Lyl	Head of household, 34 years, 1941–1975.
Brandstetter, Sebastian	Dental technician, 33 years.
Bryant, James C.	Dentist, 43 years, 1920–1963.
Burke, Richard M.	Physician, 1929–1930, left to work at Western Tuberculosis Sanatorium in Murray, Oklahoma.

Buss, Erich	Physician, arrived in 1949 as a displaced person.
Buzzelle, Leonard K.	Physician in the 1920s, left to start a private practice.
Carlson, John A.	Carpenter, 37 years.
Carroll, William Hugh	Physician, 1934–1940, died in 1940 at age 31 of a heart ailment related to rheumatic fever.
Coffman, Elena	Occupational therapist, 37 years.
Cohen, Dora	Dietician at Glen Lake and Oak Terrace, 1928–1963.
Cohen, Sumner S.	Physician, 1928–1973; medical director in 1950s.
Collins, Herbert O.	Physician and superindendent, 1915–1916, also superindentent at Minneapolis City Hospital.
Collins, James T.	Postmaster, 38 years, 1925–1963.
Crow, Earl	Chief of medical service during transition years.
Crowe, Charlotte	Student nurse in 1945; nurse, then director of nurses, 1949–1977.
Davidson, Catherine	Laundry manager, 41 years.
DeBarros, Egas	Physician, 1955, on fellowship of Rio de Janeiro, Brazil.
Delmore, Margaret	Nurse, 36 years.
Diepholz, Mary	Switchboard operator, 1971–1990, previously a TB patient.
Dietz, Hilda	Maid, 38 years.
Dragotis, D. (Jim)	Inventory clerk, 35 years.
Duncan, George R.	Physician, 1929–1936, died while at Glen Lake.
Egan, James	Baker, 34 years.
Einerson, Emma	Director of nursing education, 30+ years.
Erlanson, Oscar	Engineer, 33 years.
Faltin, James	Engineer, 30 years.
Fenger, Ejvind P.K.	Physician, 1924–1925, 1927–1955, had osteomyletis of one leg; later at Minnesota Department of Public Welfare in TB services division.
Floren, Lage	Printer, 28 years, former patient.
Forsythe, J.R.	Physician, 1952–1957.
Fraser, Lois	Sanatorium commission member, 1944–1949.
Frost, Russell	Physician, had TB as a student, Glen Lake residency in 1927, superintendent at Buena Vista 1928–1939, served in World War II, worked at the Veterans' Administration Hospital, was administrator and medical director at Glen Lake 1950–1960.
Funk, Victor K.	Physician 1926–1962, worked as a contract employee until 1977 (age seventy-eight), married Myrtle Manger, a nurse who had TB.

Gale, Edward	Sanatorium commission member, 1913–1942.
Gillard, George	Labor foreman, 34 years.
Green, Vera	Nurse, 33+ years.
Greene, Alfred	X-ray technician, 1931–1942, former patient.
Hansen, Olga	Medical secretary, 45 years.
Hanson, Richard O.	Sanatorium commission member, 1960, county commissioner.
Hardesty, W.L.	First director of the laboratory, 1926.
Harrington, Bernard	Physician, 1927–1930s.
Harrington, Francis	Consultant, Sanatorium commission member, 1937–1940.
Hastings, D.R.	Physician in outpatient clinic, 1924–1960.
Hauger, Jacob	Purchasing agent, 33 years.
Hauger, Ruth	Teacher, 25 years.
Holden, Ruth	Lab technician, 31 years.
Holmquist, Kenneth	Sanatorium commission member, 1960.
Horns, Howard L.	Sanatorium commission member, 1957–1959, physician.
Hutchinson, Dorothy	Physician, 1930–1962; came from Nopeming, where she had a University of Minnesota fellowship.
Jennings, Frank L.	Physician, 1917–1938, was a TB patient at a sanatorium in New York; left Glen Lake to work at Sunnyside Sanatorium in Indiana.
Josephs, Geri	Sanatorium commission member, 1957–1959.
Kawano, Martin M.	Physician, 1952–1953, on fellowship from Nagasaki, Japan.
King, Frances W.	Physician, 1927–1929, in China during 1930s as a university instructor, at Glen Lake again 1941–1960.
Kingman, Joseph R.	Sanatorium commission member, 1913–1942.
Kinsella, Thomas J.	Physician, 1925–1936, was a TB patient with his wife at Cragmoor in Colorado Springs, Colorado; surgeon/consultant to other sanatoriums.
Kunze, William F.	Sanatorium commission member, 1942–1944.
Kurvers, Herbert	Engineer, 30 years.
Kutcher, Edward	Pharmacist, 36 years.
Larrivee, Agnes	Night supervisor, 31 years.
Larson, Leonard M.	Physician, 1929–1960, was a doctor for Northern Pacific Railroad Hospital in Brainerd, a patient at Glen Lake for two and a half years, then joined the staff.
Law, Arthur A.	Physician, 1922–1927, performed the first lung surgery at Glen Lake, resigned because of poor health in 1927, died in 1930.

Libby, Ruby	Maid, 34 years.
Liset, Baard	Carpenter, 38 years.
Lovett, Beatrice R.	Physician, 1930–1959, worked at Hull House in Chicago before coming to Minnesota.
Lowry, Thomas	Sanitorium commission member, 1956–1957, physician.
Lundahl, Walter N.	Business manager, 1919–1947.
Lundby, W. Gerhardt	Handyman, 35 years.
Maloney, William F.	Physcian, was a patient for four years and attended medical staff meetings.
Maly, Henry W.	Physician, 1929–1934, left to work at Printers' Home Tuberculosis Hospital in Colorado Springs, Colorado.
Marcley, W.J.	Physician, first superindentent, 1916–1917, then chief of tuberculosis at the Veterans' Administration Hospital and TB consultant to the Minnesota Board of Health.
Mariette, Ernest S.	Physician, superindentent, and medical director 1916–1949, suffered a stroke and died in 1950.
Mattill, Peter M.	Physician, 1924–1957, worked at Nopeming Sanatorium and had TB before coming to Glen Lake.
Meuleners, Louise	Maid, 34 years.
Moen, Eleanor	Sanatorium commission member, 1949–1957.
Moraleda, Azarias	Physician, 1956–1957, on fellowship from the Philippines.
Morgan, Charles	Orderly, 31 years.
Naysmith, Sue	Director of nurses, 1920–1941, nurses' building named for her.
Nelson, Fred	Janitor, 31 years.
Nelson, Josephine	Laundry worker, 31 years.
Newman, Nina	Maid, 32 years.
Northrop, Cedric	Physician, 1937–1939, left to be superindentent of San Haven Sanatorium in North Dakota, was a TB control officer in the state of Washington.
Nunvar, Josephine	Laundry worker, 31 years.
Nygren, L.G.	Sanatorium commission member, 1942–1945.
Obert, Adelaide	Library clerk, 32 years.
Olsen, Trygve	Laundry washman, 30 years.
Opstad, Earl T.	Physician, 1948–1955, was a patient and stayed to be on staff.
Owinski, Joseph	Cook, 36 years.
Owinski, Martin	Cook, 25 years, brother to Joseph.

Oyama, Tsutomu	Physician, 1953–1955 on fellowship, returned to Japan to teach at the University of Hirosaki School of Medicine.
Paradis, W.G.	Physician, 1927–1929, left to be the medical director at Sunnyrest in Crookston, Minnesota.
Petter, Charles K.	Physician, 1926–1937, left to be the medical director at Lake County Sanatorium in Waukegan, Illinois.
Prazniak, John	Elevator operator, 35 years, former patient.
Pressnall, Pauline	Teacher, 32 years, married patient Louis Grenier.
Racine, Aurora	Nurse, 42 years, emigrated from Canada in 1921.
Ridler, Marguerete	Director of social service, 36 years, 1921–1957.
Rigos, F.J.	Physician, 1937–1939, fellowship through Mayo Clinic.
Roberts, Hazel	Nursing director, 29 years.
Romatko, Evelyn	Patient for 12 years, then occupational therapist for 25 years.
Rutherford, Margaret	Administrative secretary, 36 years.
Sailsbury, Charles	Painter, 30 years.
Sandell, Samuel	Physician, 1939–1944, left to work at Nopeming Sanitorium.
Schmitz, Veronica	Nurse, 30 years.
Schug, Chris	Janitor, 30 years.
Schwarting, Virginia	Bacteriologist, 1935–1964, a patient in the 1940s and again in 1962.
Schwieger, Clara	Nurse, 30 years.
Selin, Golden	Physician, 1940–1942, enlisted for World War II, worked in Michigan after discharge.
Shimek, Frank	W&S operator, 38 years.
Siegel, Clarence	Physician, 1930–1940, medical director at Otter Tail Sanatorium, back to Glen Lake until 1945, left to establish a private practice.
Skeffington, Hilda	Cook, 30 years.
Smith, Leslie	Laboratory technician, 1928–1973, Glen Lake/Oak Terrace.
Song, Ho-Seung	Physician, 1955, on fellowship, medical school professor in Korea.
Stenseth, Jeanette	Nurse, 32 years.
Steward, James	Maintenance foreman, 36 years.
Strader, Ernest	Physician, 1931–1933, resigned because of ill health, died 1934.
Stubben, Owen	Administrator, 1960–1961, until transition to state nursing home.
Tomsche, Edward	Engineer, 31 years.

Townsend, Lucille	Director of household, 1916–1941, Townsend Hall named for her.
Trytten, Edwin G.	Physician, 1943, served in World War II, at Glen Lake again 1945–1946, left to work for the Veterans' Administration in Duluth and Michigan.
Tsai, Shih H.	Physician, 1947–1959, from Japan, continued at Oak Terrace and Veterans' Administration Hospital as a radiologist; his wife, Ruby, worked at Glen Lake as a nurses' aide.
Twomey, John E.	Sanatorium commission member, 1960, physician.
VanWinkle, Charlotte	Physician, 1925–1935, pathologist and laboratory director.
Vosmek, August	Maintenance engineer, 40 years.
Walker, Mrs. Walter	Sanatorium commission member, 1960
Washburn, Helen	Clerk, 31+ years.
White, S. Marx	Sanatorium commission member, 1919–1937, 1940–1955.
Wiegert, Velma	Nurse, 40+ years.
Williams, Fred	Engineer, 33 years.
Wilweding, Carl	Bookkeeper, 31 years, former patient.
Wright, Raymond	Sanatorium commission member, 1945–1959.
Ylvisaker, Anna	Operating room supervisor, 35 years, 1927–1962.
Yue, Wen-Yao	Physician, 1954–1962, arrived from China, continued as consultant at Glen Lake/Oak Terrace after transition.

Sources: Board of Hennepin County Commissioners, letter to author, January 18, 1990; medical staff, meeting ,inutes; Glen Lake Sanatorium pamphlet, 1960.

Appendix B
Minnesota's State and County Sanatoriums

Name	City	Post-Sanatorium Era
Ah-gwah-ching	Walker	Converted to a state-owned nursing home in 1962 and operated as such until 2008. It was added to the National Register of Historic Places in 2001, but all buildings except for a gazebo were demolished in 2010. Records are at the Minnesota Historical Society.
Buena Vista	Wabasha	Converted to Buena Vista Rest Home in 1956, and most of the buildings were later demolished. Records are at the Minnesota Historical Society.
Deerwood	Deerwood	Converted to Cedar Brook Manor in 1952. Since the nursing home closed in the 1970s, the site has been used for a skating rink and hockey camp.
Fair Oaks Lodge	Wadena	Converted to Shady Lane Rest Home in 1952. The main building is part of the Fair Oaks Lodge retirement community.
Glen Lake	Oak Terrace/ Minnetonka	Converted to Oak Terrace Nursing Home in 1961, with the last TB patient on census in 1976. Buildings were demolished in 1993. Two summer camp buildings remain with National Register of Historic Places status. Records are at the Minnesota Historical Society.
Lake Julia	Pupoksy	Converted to Lake Julia Rest Home in 1954; one building still stands unoccupied on private property. A few records are at the Minnesota Historical Society.
Mineral Springs	Cannon Falls	Used as an adolscent treatment center and vacated in the 1980s. Buildings were torn down in the 1990s for housing development. A few records are at the Minnesota Historical Society.

Nopeming	Nopeming/ Duluth	The Trudeau Building converted to Trudeau Nursing Home Unit in 1957; the campus became Nopeming Nursing Home in 1971. The facility closed in 2002. The buildings stand vacant as of 2016, and the main building was the subject of a *Ghost Hunters* episode on the Travel Channel. Records are at the Minnesota Historical Society and the University of Minnesota–Duluth.
Oakland Park	Thief River Falls	In 1954, patients were transferred Sunnrest Sanatorium in Crookston, and the building was converted to Oakland Park Nursing Home in 1955. After a new building was constructed for the nursing home, the old one served as a dormitory for students and then was unoccupied for several years. It was torn down in 1999.
Otter Tail	Battle Lake	Converted to Otter Tail County Nursing Home in 1955; as Golden Living Center, it closed in 2012. The sanatorium cemetery has some unmarked graves. A few records are at the Otter Tail County Historical Society.
Ramsey	St. Paul	The county pavilion at Ancker Hospital was converted to a pediatrics ward in 1951. The building was razed in the 1960s. The children's preventorium at Lake Owasso closed in 1953. Some records are at the Minnesota Historical Society.
Riverside	Granite Falls	Closed in the 1960s, with an outpatient clinic operating in Granite Falls. The building became Turnabout House in 1970 for chemical dependency treatment. Buildings were razed in the 1990s. Records are at the Minnesota Historical Society.
Sand Beach	Lake Park	Converted to Sunnyside Rest Home, with original buildings eventually torn down. The Sunnyside Care Center operates on the same site.
Southwest	Worthington	Closed in 1957 and sold to Southwestern Minnesota Crippled Children's Hospital-School, Inc. Later renamed the Lakeview School, in operated from 1958 until 1996. Records are at the Minnesota Historical Society.
Sunnyrest	Crookston	Closed in 1957, except for an outpatient clinic, which closed in 1977. Some records are at the Minnesota Historical Society.

Notes

Prologue

[1]Frederick Manfred, interview by author, August 19, 1990, videocassette, Minneton-ka, MN.

Chapter 1

[1]"Twenty Years Ago, in Howling Snow Storm, Glen Lake Sanatorium Admitted First Patient." *Minneapolis Tribune*, January 1936. Also, Minnesota Historical Society, Glen Lake Sanatorium patient records, 1903-1925.

[2]*Terrace Topics*, June 1945.

[3]"Tuberculosis Hospital at Glen Lake Will be Opened on Tuesday, Inside Ward Not Yet Complete." *Minneapolis Morning Tribune*, January 1, 1916.

[4]*Hippocrates, Of the epidemics.* Book I, Section 1, First Constitution, 2. Tr. by Francis Adams.

[5]Edward Hayes, *Tuberculosis as it comes and goes.* Springfield, IL: Charles C. Thom-as, 1943), 7.

[6]Godias J. Drolet, "Present trends of case fatality rates in tuberculosis." *American Review of Tuberculosis*, February 1938. 37, 2:125-151.

[7]Ernest Mariette, "Your Questions – Answered here." *Terrace Topics*, January 1943, 4.

[8]Jared Diamond, *Guns, Germs, and Steel.* (New York: W. W. Norton & Co., 1997). Diamond devotes a chapter to the "Lethal Gift of Livestock" and how this "sinister gift" contributed to the big advantage that Europeans had over the non-European peoples they conquered.

[9]Jane E. Buikstra, *Prehistoric Tuberculosis in the Americas.* (Northwestern University Archaeological Program, Scientific papers, 1981), 1-5.

[10]Jane Buikstra, *Tuberculosis in the Americas.* (Northwestern University Archeologi-cal Program, Scientific Papers, 1981), 12.

[11]Paul Farmer, *Infections and Inequalities: The Modern Plagues.* (Berkeley: University of California Press, 1999), 202.

[12]Roy W. Meyer, *History of the Santee Sioux.* (Lincoln: University of Nebraska Press, 1967), 68.

[13]Samuel William Pond, *The Dakota Sioux in Minnesota as They Were in 1834.* (Minnesota Historical Society Collections). Quoted in J. Arthur Myers, Invited and Conquered: Historical Sketch of Tuberculosis in Minnesota. (St. Paul: Webb Publishing, 1949).

[14]Williams, ed. *The Minnesota Guide.* (St. Paul: E.H. Burritt & Co., 1869.)

[15]J.W. McClung, *Minnesota as it is in 1870.* (St. Paul: the author, 1870).

[16]Lucy Leavenworth Wilder Morris, ed., *Old Rail Fence Corners: Frontier Tales told by Minnesota pioneers.* (St. Paul: Minnesota Historical Society Press, 1976). Reprint of the 2nd edition of *Old Rail Fence Corners: The A.B.C.'s of Minnesota History,* (Austin, MN: F.H. McCulloch Print Co., 1915).

[17]Brewer Mattocks, Minnesota as a Home for Invalids. (Philadelphia: J.B. Lippincott Co., 1881), 147.

[18]F. Scott Fitzgerald, "Minnesota's Capital in the Role of Main Street" in Matthew Joseph Broccoli, Judith Baughman, *F. Scott Fitzgerald on Authorship,* (University of South Carolina Press, 1996), 81.

[19]J. Arthur Myers, *Invited and Conquered: Historical Sketch of Tuberculosis in Minnesota.* (St. Paul: Webb Publishing), 23.

[20]F.B. Sanborn, ed., *The Writings of Henry David Thoreau,* VI, Familiar Letters. (Boston: Houghton Mifflin; 1906), 383-84.

[21]Sanborn, 390-91.

[22]Sanborn, 393.

[23]J.F. Williams, ed., *The Minnesota Guide.* (St. Paul: E.H. Burritt & Co., 1869).

[24]William Mayo, presidential address to Minnesota State Medical Association, 1873, quoted by J. Arthur Myers in "Entrance, Rise and Fall of Tuberculosis in Minnesota," *Minnesota Medicine,* September 1977, 679.

[25]Theodore C. Blegen, *Minnesota: A History of the State.* (University of Minnesota Press, 1963), 198.

[26]Myers, *Invited and Conquered,* 15.

[27]Ibid., 83.

[28]*First Annual Report of the State Board of Health of Minnesota.* January 1873. 42.

[29]Myers, *Invited and Conquered,* 82-83.

[30]"Sanitary History of Tuberculosis in Minneapolis," *Annual Reports of the Various City Officers of the City of Minneapolis, Minnesota.* (1907), 385.

[31]Myers, *Invited and Conquered,* 101.

[32]Ibid., 519. Dr. Frost's grandson, Russell, would contract tuberculosis as an intern and later serve as a medical director at two sanatoriums in Minnesota.

[33]Ethel McClure, *More than a Roof: The Development of Minnesota Poor Farms and Homes for the Aged.* (St. Paul: Minnesota Historical Society, 1968), 03.

[34]Ibid., 104. Also, "An Unlamented Era: County Poor Farms in Minnesota." *Minnesota History,* December 1963, 365.

[35]Myers, *Invited and Conquered,* 115, 116.

Chapter 2

[1]Silesia was part of Germany at the time. Following the Potsdam Agreement of 1945, it was transferred to Poland.

[2]Thomas Mann, John Woods tr., *Magic Mountain* (Everyman's Library, 2005).

[3]J.A. Myers, *Invited and Conquered* (St. Paul: Webb Publishing Co., 1949), 23.

[4]Edward Hayes, *Tuberculosis as It Comes and Goes* (Springfield, IL: Bannerstone House, 1947, 2nd ed.) Thomas M. Daniel in *The History of Tuberculosis* credits Joseph Gleitsman with opening the United States' first sanatorium in Asheville, North Carolina. And although not considered a formal sanatorium, it's likely that the first institution in the United States for the care of the tuberculous was the Channing Street Home for Sick and Destitute Women in Boston's Federal Street Church, opened by Harriet Ryan in 1857. Channing provided lodging for women terminally ill with consumption. Source: Kass, Amalie M. "A Brief History of the Channing Laboratory."

[5]"He Says Sanitarium – I say Sanatorium' – So What?" *Terrace Topics*, April 1944.

[6]*Tuberculosis Hospital and Sanatorium Directory*. New York: National Tuberculosis Association, 1951).

[7]Myers, *Invited and Conquered*, 97.

[8]Henry Longstreet Taylor, "The necessity of special institutions for the consumptive poor," *Northwestern Lancet*, 1893, xiii, 469-473.

[9]Myers, *Invited and Conquered*, 108.

[10]Ibid., 398.

[11]Ibid., 398.

[12]Ibid., 486.

[13]Jerry Vessels, "Building our sanatoriums," *Everybody's Health*, 1956, June, July, August, 8.

[14]Jerry Vessels. "Building Our Sanatoriums," *Everybody's Health*, July, August, 1956: 9. Also, "Serious work of society women," *Minneapolis Morning Tribune*. Feb. 28, 1909: 13, and "Illustrations showing G. H. Christian Hospital for little victims of the awful white plague." *Minneapolis Tribune*, July 29, 1906: 15. Both retrieved from ProQuest Historical Newspapers.

[15]"Disease menace is lifting from city; Miss Patterson recounts war for health." *Minneapolis Morning Tribune*, January 18, 1920, sec. B.

[16]"George H. Christian further outlines plans for Minneapolis consumption hospital." *Minneapolis Tribune*, July 14, 1906, 7. Retrieved from ProQuest Historical Newspapers.

[17]*Hudson's Dictionary of Minneapolis*, 1908, 52. Also, *History of Minneapolis, Gateway to the Northwest*, Rev. Marion Daniel Shutter, ed. Vol. 1, (Minneapolis: S.J. Clarke Publishing Company, 1923) 511.

[18]"Hopewell Hospital to Open," *Minneapolis Morning Tribune*, September 6, 1908, 6.

[19]"Where are Red Cross stamps, ask women," *Minneapolis Morning Tribune*, December 13, 1908, 11.

[20]Myers, *Invited and Conquered*, 409. Piney Ridge at Jenkins, MN, was built by Dr. J. H. Sandberg in 1901 as a fishing resort for fellow physicians. He converted it to a sanatorium with 12 cabins and 13 floored tents, but by 1911 it was again operating strictly as a resort.

[21]Henry M. Bracken, *Health Department Correspondence*, Minnesota Historical Society Archives.

Chapter 3

[1]Hennepin County Sanatorium Commission, Glen Lake Sanatorium, 1961, 14.

[2]"Tuberculosis Hospital at Glen Lake Will be Opened on Tuesday. Inside ward not yet complete." *Minneapolis Morning Tribune*, January 1, 1916, 16. Also, "County sanatorium gets first patients," *The Minneapolis Journal*, January 6, 1916.

[3]"Fighting the white plague," *Minneapolis Morning Tribune*, August 6, 1916, sec. E.

[4]J. Arthur Myers, Invited and Conquered: Historical Sketch of Tuberculosis in Minnesota, (St. Paul: Webb Publishing Co., 1949) 105.

[5]Thomas Spees Carrington, *Tuberculosis Hospital and Sanatorium Construction*, (New York: National Association for the Study and Prevention of Tuberculosis, 1911, 27, 76.

[6]Carrington, 14.

[7]Carrington, 19.

[8]Minnesota Department of Health, Health Department Correspondence, in Minnesota Historical Society archives.

[9]Frank L. Jennings, "From Fifty to Seven Hundred . . ." *Terrace Topics* VI, no. 3 (1938): 5. Also Terrace Topics IX (1941): 16.

[10]*Hennepin County Medical Center, Ambulance Service History*. Retrieved June 21, 2010. <http://www.hcmc.org/education/ems/ems_dept/ambulance/history.htm.> [no longer valid] The ambulance service stopped in 1923.

[11]Ceil Robertson Marshall and Marion Stewart, *The Glen Lake Area*, 1982. The library at the Minnesota Historical Society is named in honor of the Gale family.

[12]Jennings, Frank L., "Know Your San," *Terrace Topics* I, no. 2 (1933): 2, 3.

[13]Carrington, 27. The references are to the Tuberculosis Hospital in Washington, D.C. and the Georgia State Sanatorium in Alto, GA, at which "Negro quarters which are to be practically the same as those provided for the white patients, but entirely separated from them and concealed by a thick growth of trees and shrubbery."

[14]Nichols, a railroad porter, admitted on November, 14, 1916, died on May 5, 1917.

[15]Lucile R. Townsend, "Our household, past and present," *Terrace Topics* 2 (1933).

[16]"Lucille Townsend," ownsend, *Terrace Topics*, IX, no. 3 (1941): 4.

[17]Hennepin County Tuberculosis Association, Average Length of Stay. Glen Lake Sanatorium Patients, 1951.

[18]"Glen Lake Sanitarium [sic], Opened Two Months Ago, Already Housing 48 Tubercular Patients," *Minneapolis Morning Tribune*, March 12, 1916, sec. B. Margaret Kelley was discharged as "Improved" on April 24, 1916. Glen Lake Sanatorium patient records 1903-1925, MNHS.

[19]"Looking Back," *Terrace Topics*, I, no. 6 (1934): 12.

[20]Oletta Desmond, "Walker in 1916." *Terrace Topics* I, no. 8 (1934). Oletta, a widow, came to Glen Lake from Ah-gwah-ching. Her sons lived with relatives.

[21]Jennings, "From Fifty to Seven Hundred . . ." 5.

[22]*Davidson's Minneapolis Directory*, 1915. Advertisement, 2399.

[23]"Glen Lake Sanitarium [sic], Opened Two Months Ago, Already Housing 48 Tubercular Patients," *Minneapolis Morning Tribune*, March 12, 1916, sec. B. Also, Frank L. Jennings, "The Permeability of Paper Sputum Napkins," *The American*

Review of Tuberculosis. XXXII, no. 3, (1935): 304. Also, Frank L. Jennings, "Factors Contributing to the Further Reduction of Tuberculous Infection," *Minnesota Medicine,* 18 (1935): 280.

[24]Herbert A. Burns, *Procedure and Technic,* Ah-gwah-ching (1937).

[25]"Glen Lake Sanitarium [sic], Opened Two Months Ago, Already Housing 48 Tubercular Patients," sec. B.

[26]"Glen Lake Sanatorium Like 'Home, Sweet Home'; The Phonograph Arrives," *Minneapolis Morning Tribune,* March 24, 1916, 10. The price of a standard VVX phonograph would have been about $100 at the time, the equivalent of $2,100 in 2012 dollars. The Minnesota Loan and Trust Company, at 311 Nicollet Avenue, was a predecessor of Norwest Bank, later Wells Fargo.

[27]"Invalided by White Plague, He Becomes a Silhouet [sic] Artist," *Minneapolis Morning Tribune,* September 17, 1916, 12. Two other Pugsley children died shortly after their births in 1909 and 1914. Other sources: Patient and census records, MNHS.

[28]*Minnesota Death Certificates.*

[29]*Terrace Topics,* XII, no. 10. (1945).

[30]"Fighting the White Plague," *Minneapolis Morning Tribune,* August 6, 1916, sec. E.

[31]*Minneapolis City Directory,* U. S. Census records, marriage and death certificates. MNHS.

[32]*Terrace Topics.* VI, no. 2 (1933): 4.

Chapter 4

[1]Lucile Townsend, "Our Household – past and present," *Terrace Topics.* (1933).

[2]*A Directory of Sanatoriums, Hospitals and Day Camps for the Treatment of Tuberculosis in the United States* (New York: National Tuberculosis Association, 1919). Also, <http://www.pinecogen.org/Pokegama%20Sanatorium.html> retrieved Sept. 19, 2013.

[3]George Grimm, "Little Store is Big Thing to Glen Lake," *Minneapolis Tribune,* December 16, 1949. Also, patient records and 1930 federal census, MNHS. Grenier married the Sanatorium's schoolteacher, Pauline, and he died in 1951. "Polly Pressnall reminisces about teaching at Glen Lake Sanatorium," Minnetonka Sailor, September 14, 1981, Sec. A, 1.

[4]Myers, *Invited and Conquered,* 426-428. Also, "Dorothy Walton Named to Social Service Work," *Minneapolis Morning Tribune,* February 17, 1918, 12.

[5]Townsend, "Our Household."

[6]"Lenore Ward to Take Up Task of Dorothy Walton," *Minneapolis Morning Tribune,* July 25, 1918, 6. Miss Ward's name was given as Lenora, Lenore, and Lanore in various newspaper articles and in Myers' book. Records in Ancestry.com have it listed as Lanore.

[7]"Patients at Glen Lake to Enjoy Film Program," *Minneapolis Morning Tribune,* October 24, 1919, 10. Also, the movie was probably *Missing Husband* (no's'), a one-reel, 10-minute short from Universal Films produced in 1919. *Missing Husbands* (with an 's') was a seven-reel French film made in 1921. *Royal Nymphs* not found in a database. Source: Robert DeFlores, film archivist and historian. Telephone conversation with the author. July 19, 2012.

[8]Myers, *Invited and Conquered*, 219.

[9]Esmond R. Long, "Tuberculosis," *Preventive Medicine in World War II*, Volume IV, Medical Department, United States Army. <<http://history.amedd.army.mil/booksdocs/wwii/PM4/DEFAULT.htm.>> Retrieved April 7, 2014.

[10]Myers, *Invited and Conquered*, 469.

[11]"War on Disease Plagues," *Minneapolis Morning Tribune*, March 27, 1919, 16.

[12]Godias Drolet, "World War I and Tuberculosis," *American Journal of Public Health*, 35 (1945): 690.

[13]*Twenty-five years of Fighting Tuberculosis in Minneapolis and Hennepin County, 1903-1928* (Minneapolis: Hennepin County Tuberculosis Association), 48.

[14]Myers, *Invited and Conquered*, 416. Also, The Hennepin Commonhealth, 2 (1920).

[15]"Hospitals to Show Work of Patients which Helps Cure," *Minneapolis Morning Tribune*, April 25, 1920, sec. D. Mrs. George Chase (Carolyn) Christian was the daughter-in-law of George H. and Lenore Christian. Her husband had died shortly after his parents, and she assumed their charitable roles. Mrs. Kingman's husband was a member of the tuberculosis commission, and Mrs. Sumner McKnight's husband was a prominent Minneapolis businessman, brother to Carolyn Christian.

[16]Myers, *Invited and Conquered*, 243.

[17]*Terrace Topics*, I, no. 6 (1934): 12.

[18]"What are We Here For?" *The Arrow*. 1, no. 6, (1921).

[19]*Trudeau School of Tuberculosis, Historic Saranac Lake*<http://localwiki.net/hsl/Trudeau_School_of_Tuberculosis>> retrieved September 21, 2013.

[20]"Entertainments and Decorations will Bring Christmas Cheer to Minneapolis Hospitals," *Minneapolis Morning Tribune*, December 20, 1920, 10.

[21]Hall, Pearl M. "Beds for the Tuberculous," *Minneapolis Morning Tribune*, January 31, 1917, 6.

[22]"Phthisis Fight May Be Aided $350,000," *Minneapolis Morning Tribune*, January 18, 1917, 4.

[23]"$300,000 Asked for Fight upon Tuberculosis," *Minneapolis Morning Tribune*, December 26, 1920, 12.

[24]"Sanatorium Contract Awarded," *Minneapolis Morning Tribune*, December 8, 1918, sec. A. Klarquist and Sons also worked on the Great Northern Railroad depot, the Roosevelt Community Library, the Farmers Terminal Packing Plant at Red Rock and several state institutional buildings. Mr. Klarquist died suddenly in 1920 at forty years of age. His son died two months later. Arthur Dunham and Engelbret Sund formed the Sund & Dunham architectural firm in 1911. During their partnership, they were responsible for designing schools, churches and institutions in the Minneapolis and St. Paul area and also the Moose Lake State Hospital and buildings at Ah-gwah-ching.

[25]"Health Officials Inspect Glen Lake Sanatorium at Opening of New Building," *Minneapolis Morning Tribune*, April 23, 1921, 29.

[26]"Trivia," *Terrace Topics*, June 1946.

[27]Hospital Inspection Report, Fire Marshal Division, Department of Public Safety, State of Minnesota, 1965. MNHS archives.

[28]Ernest Mariette, "Prevention of Tuberculosis among Nursing and Auxiliary Personnel," *The American Journal of Nursing*, 46, no.12, (1946): 825-827. Retrieved from JSTOR, September 7, 2008.

[29]Hennepin County Sanatorium Commission. Glen Lake Sanatorium Report, 1926, 8.

[30]Charlotte Crowe, interview by author, videocassette, 1990, Minnetonka, MN. Author collection.

Chapter 5

[1]Frances M. Pottenger, *Tuberculosis and How to Combat It: A Book for the Patient* (St. Louis: C.V. Mosby Company, 1921), 65.

[2]J. Harry Bendes, "Heliotherapy in Tuberculosis" (paper presented at the annual meeting of the American Sanatorium Association at Oak Terrace, MN, June 16, 1925). MNHS Archives.

[3]"Fighting the White Plague with Old Sol's Rays at Glen Lake," *Minneapolis Morning Tribune*, June 19, 1921, sec. C.

[4]Alexandra V. Yamshchikov, et al. "Vitamin D status and antimicrobial peptide cathelicidin (LL-37) concentrations in patients with active pulmonary tuberculosis," *American Journal of Clinical Nutrition*, 92 (2010): 603-611. Also M. Nathaniel Mead, "Benefits of Sunlight : A Bright Spot for Human Health," *Environmental Health Perspectives*, 116 (2008): A160-A167. Retrieved June 15, 2014 from <<http://www.ncbi.nlm.nih.gov/pmc/articles/PMC2290997/>>.

[5]Bernard Langdon Wyatt, "Limitations of Heliotherapy in pulmonary tuberculosis," *Annals of Internal Medicine*, 4 (1930): 376-378.

[6]Arthur J. Myers. *Tuberculosis among Children and Young Adults* (Springfield, IL: Charles C. Thomas, 1951).

[7]*Excelsior-Minnetonka Record*, November 24, 1922.

[8]Norma Anderson, ed. "Delois Anderson Clair," in *San Memories* (n.p., 1990), 16.

[9]Bendes, "Heliotherapy in tuberculosis."

[10]*The Arrow*, 1, no. 6 (1921).

[11]Bendes, "Heliotherapy in tuberculosis."

[12]"Like the sun," *Terrace Topics*, III, no. 19 (1937): 4

[13]Al Greene, "The Song of the Buy-o," *Terrace Topics*, (1941).

[14]"It Used to be Hennco," *Terrace Topics*, III, no. 7 (1936): 7.

[15]"More Room Needed for Sufferers from White Plague; $1,500,000 Asked for Addition to Sanitarium," *Minneapolis Morning Tribune*, January 30, 1921, 16.

[16]"Ceremony Arranged for Signing of Bill to Aid Sanatorium," *Minneapolis Morning Tribune*, March 28, 1921, 3. Carl Wilwerding did leave Glen Lake and died in 1955.

[17]Myers, *Invited and Conquered*, 155.

[18]"Christmas Seals to Help Keep Others from Margie's Plight," *Minneapolis Star*, November 13, 1926.

[19]Emile Berliner, Muddy Jim and Other Rhymes; 12 Illustrated Health Jingles for Children (Washington D.C., 1929) 5. << http://loc.gov. >> Retrieved July 17, 2013.

[20]"Trudeau Elementary School." *Marshall/Marshall University High School Alumni Newsletter*, 19, no 1 (2011). The Thomas School was renamed Trudeau Elementary School in 1913. <<https://diversity.umn.edu/disability/sites/diversity.umn.edu. disability/files/MHS%20January%202011%20Alumni%20News.pdf> > Retrieved 11/17/2013.

[21]Myers, *Invited and Conquered*, 407. Also, Leonard Wilson, "Medical Revolution in Minnesota: A History of the University of Minnesota Medical School" (St. Paul: Midewiwin Press, 1989):332 and "Lymanhurst Donor Lauds City's Program," *Minneapolis Morning Tribune*, January 15, 1922, sec. A.

[22]Patricia D'Antonio, et al. *Nurses' Work: Issues across Time and Place*. (New York: Springer Publishing Co., 2007).

[23]Myers, *Invited and Conquered*, 410. The preventorium closed in 1953 and reopened in 1955 as Lake Owasso Children's Home.

[24]"Board Responsibility for Open-Air School Plan of Committee; Anti-Tuberculosis Body Wants to Devote Energy to Other Work," *Minneapolis Morning Tribune*, February 20, 1916, 11.

[25]"Funeral Services for George H. Christian to be Held Tomorrow," *Minneapolis Morning Tribune*, January 20, 1916, 10.

[26]"Benjamin Reports on Anti-phthisis Work," *Minneapolis Morning Tribune*, November 3, 1918, sec. C.

[27]"$300,000 Asked for Fight upon Tuberculosis," *Minneapolis Morning Tribune*, December 26, 1920, 12.

[28]Sanatorium for Child Patients Formally Opens," *Minneapolis Morning Tribune*, May 14, 1922, 8.

[29]Virginia Dustin, "Glen Lake Children's Hospital: Sick Children Made Well and Happy Again," *Golfer and Sportsman*, 1947, 6.

[30]"Betty Carroll, interview, videocassette, 1990, Minnetonka, MN. Author collection.

[31]"The Keyhole Employee," *Terrace Topics*, December 1937. Also, Norma Anderson, ed. "Virginia Schwarting" in *San Memories* (n.p., 1990): 58.

[32]"The Doghouse," *Terrace Topics*, December 1936, 5.

Chapter 6

[1]Francis M. Pottenger, *Tuberculosis and How to Combat It: A Book for the Patient*. (St. Louis: C.V. Mosby Company): 199, 201, 207.

[2]Fred G. Holmes, *Tuberculosis: A Book for the Patient*. (New York: D. Appleton-Century Co., 1935) 88,89.

[3]*Excelsior-Minnetonka Record*, November 24, 1922.

[4]*Medical Staff Meeting Minutes*, Glen Lake Sanatorium. MNHS Archives.

[5]Ernest Mariette. "Localized Rest in the Treatment of Pulmonary Tuberculosis," *American Review of Tuberculosis*, XI, no. 1, (1924).

[6]*Information and Rules for Patients at Glen Lake Sanatorium*, Oak Terrace, Minn. (Oak Terrace, MN: Glen Lake Sanatorium Print Shop, 1935).

[7]Helen Hanson, interview, August 19, 1990, videocassette, Minnetonka, MN.

[8]Beatrice Olson, letter, January 17, 1983.

[9]Frances Lange, interview, July 9, 2010, audiocassette, Bloomington, MN. Author collection.

[10]*Medical Staff Meeting Minutes*, October 21, 1940.

[11]Norma Anderson, ed. "Howard Johnson" in *San Memories* (n.p., 1990).

[12]Norma Anderson, ed. "Anonymous" in *San Memories* (n.p. 1990): 22.

[13]Frances Melby, telephone interview, June 2013, transcript. Author collection. Ruby was at the San for about five years and died there in 1937.

[14]*Medical Staff Meeting Minutes*, April 11, 1927.

[15]Norma Anderson, ed. 1990. "Deloise Anderson Clair" in San Memories (n.p. 1990): 16.

[16]Ernest Mariette, "Question Box," *Terrace Topics*, (1941) 8.

[17]"Pick-ups," *Terrace Topics*, July 1935.

[18]Norma Anderson, ed. "Esther Giere Johnson" in *San Memories* (n.p. 1990): 74.

[19]Maryann Shorba, Diary. Excerpts from January 24, February 10, March 17, April 27, and April 30, 1940. Freya Manfred collection.

[20]Huseboe, Arthur R. and Nancy Owen Nelson, eds. *The Selected Letters of Frederick Manfred, 1932-1954*. (Lincoln: University of Nebraska Press, 1989): 115. Letter to John Huizenga, January 19, 1941.

[21]Lisa Diedrich, *Treatments: Language, Politics, and the Culture of Illness* (Minneapolis: University of Minnesota Press, 2007): 3.

[22]Pottenger, *Tuberculosis and How to Combat It*, 198.

[23]Sadie Fuller Seagrave, *Saints' Rest* (St. Louis: C.V. Mosby, 1918). Also, Ancestry. com. Seagrave was born in Minnesota in 1882. Her husband Amos, whom she married in 1906, died of TB in 1910. Seagrave spent time at other sanatoriums, including Iowa State Sanatorium in Oakdale. She passed away in 1972.

[24]*Information and Rules for Patients at Glen Lake Sanatorium*, Oak Terrace, Minn.

[25]"Question Box," *Terrace Topics*, January 1942, p.12.

[26]Norma Anderson, ed. "Esther Giere Johnson" 69.

[27]Norma Anderson, ed. "Deloise Anderson Clair," 18.

[28]William H. Carroll, "Habits and Tuberculous." *Terrace Topics*, May 1939, pp. 3,11,23.

[29]Frederick Feikema Manfred, interview, August 9,1990, videocassette. Author collection.

[30]Geoffrey C. Bowker and Susan L. Star, *Sorting Things Out: Classification and its Consequences* (MIT Press, 1999).

[31]Julius Roth, *Timetables: Structuring the Passage of Time in Hospital Treatment and Other Careers* (New York: Bobbs-Merrill, 1963): xv, xvi, 75.

[32]Ernest Mariette, *Report of a Year's Activities of Glen Lake Sanatorium*. (Paper presented at a joint meeting of the Hennepin County Medical Society and the Women's Auxiliary, Oak Terrace, MN, November 1, 1926).

[33]Ernest Mariette, "How Sanatorium patients are admitted and their daily schedule," *Modern Hospital*, XXVIII, no. 5 (1927).

[34]Roth, *Timetables*.

[35]*Terrace Topics*, November 1934.

Chapter 7

[1]Peter M. Mattill, "Question Box," *Terrace Topics*, November 1935, 14.

[2]Milton Rosenblatt, "Pulmonary Tuberculosis: Evolution of Modern Therapy." *Bulletin of the New York Academy of Medicine*. 49, no.3 (1971). Also, Myers, Invited and Conquered, 65.

[3]Ernest Mariette, "Question Box," *Terrace Topics*, IX, no. 3 (1941): 8.

[4]P. Bergeron, "Pneumo Then and Now," *Terrace Topics*, June 1937, 3.

[5]Edward Hayes, *Tuberculosis as It Comes and Goes*. (Springfield Il: Charles C. Thomas, 1943).

[6]Zdenek Hrubec, John D. Boice, Jr., Richard R. Monson, et al. "Breast Cancer after Multiple Chest Fluoroscopies," *Cancer Research*. 1989; 49:229-234

[7]Norma Anderson, ed. "Dora Cohen" in *San Memories* (n.p., 1990) 63.

[8]Thomas J. Kinsella, "Pneumothorax Evaluated," *Terrace Topics*. February 1936. 4.

[9]Victor Funk, interview, 1990, videocassette, author collection. Also, Charles Sampson, Agriculture, engineering, buildings, and grounds report. (Glen Lake Sanatorium, 1943) MNHS Archives.

[10]Ernest Mariette, Localized rest in the treatment of tuberculosis (Paper read before the Clinical Section at the annual meeting of the National Tuberculosis Association, Atlanta, GA, May 1924). MNHS Archives.

[11]Edward Hayes, 108.

[12]Ernest Mariette, Extrapleural Thoracoplasty (Paper presented to the staff of Lymanhurst, Minneapolis, MN. March 13, 1923). The surgeon was Dr. Carl Hedblom.

[13]Myers, *Invited and Conquered*, 144.

[14]Norma Anderson, ed. "Beatrice Olson," in *San Memories*, (n.p, 1990) 20.

[15]"San Jottings," *Terrace Topics*, November 1935, 13.

[16]"Mystic Order of the Short Rib," *Terrace Topics*, October 1938, 6.

[17]Myers, *Invited and Conquered*, 129.

[18]"The danger of swallowing sputum," *Terrace Topics*, August 1944.

[19]*Head Nurses Meeting Minutes*, Glen Lake Sanatorium, July 1, 1940, MNHS Archives. Also, "Sanatorium Facts," *Terrace Topics*, January 1942.

[20]Frank Lane, "The Guinea Pig and Tuberculosis," *Terrace Topics*, December 1936. 6.

[21]Leslie Smith, interview with Colleen Spadaccini,1990, videocassette, author collection.

[22]Norma Anderson, "Robert Engstrom" in *San Memories* (n.p.,1990) 9, 10.

[23]*Medical Staff Meeting Minutes*, September 28, 1931.

[24]*Medical Staff Meeting Minutes*, October 19, 1931.

[25]Barbara Bates, *Bargaining for Life: A Social History of Tuberculosis, 1876-1938* (Philadelphia: University of Pennsylvania Press,1992) 298.

[26]Statistical reports of Glen Lake Sanatorium in the Minnesota History Center archives.

[27]Mark Caldwell, *The Last Crusade: The War on Consumption, 1862-1954*, 1988 (New York: Atheneum), 256.

Chapter 8

[1]"In Memoriam," *Terrace Topics*, VIII, no. 10 (1941). Her children also donated Jewish books.

[2]Edward W. Hayes, *Tuberculosis as It Comes and Goes*, 2nd ed. (Springfield, IL: Charles C. Thomas, 1947) 178.

[3]Will Ross, *I Wanted to Live* (Wisconsin Anti-tuberculosis Association, 1953) 95.

[4]Beatrice Olson, interview, January 17, 1983, author's collection.

[5]Lucille Steinhagen Faucher, interview, May 30, 2013, audiocassette transcript, author's collection.

[6]*Medical Staff Meeting Minutes*, October 26, 1925. MNHS Archives.

[7]"Gossip column (1W)." *Terrace Topics*, Oct. 1943. Pp.17,18. Also, Terrace Topics, Oct. 1943.

[8]Maryanna Shorba, diary, January 18, 1940.

[9]Norma Anderson, ed. "Esther Johnson" in *San Memories*, (n.p., 1990) 75.

[10]Arthur R. Husboe and Nancy Owen Nelson, eds., *Selected Letters of Frederick Manfred, 1932-1954* (Lincoln: University of Nebraska Press, 1988) 259.

[11]Manuel Martinez, interview by author, November 3, 2001, audiocassette, author's collection.

[12]Delores Romatko Farr, interview, 1990, videocassette, author's collection.

[13]*Medical Staff Meeting Minutes*. March 5, 1928, and Nov 16, 1942.

[14]*Medical Staff Meeting Minutes*, Dec. 5, 1949.

[15]Ernest S. Mariette, *Problems of the Sanatorium Administrator* (paper presented to the Mississippi Valley Sanatorium Association, Dayton, Ohio, Sept. 24, 1937).

[16]*Medical Staff Meeting Minutes*, Jan 23, 1933.

[17]*Medical Staff Meeting Minutes*, July 24, 1933.

[18]*Medical Staff Meeting Minutes*, November 27, 1933.

[19]*Medical Staff Meeting Minutes*, December 18, 1933.

[20]*Medical Staff Meeting Minutes*, March 13, 1933.

[21]*Report of the Glen Lake Sanatorium, 1932-33* (Oak Terrace, MN: Glen Lake Sanatorium Vocational School) 38.

[22]"Bio Brevities: From Paint Pot to Palette," *Terrace Topics*, June 1937. P.12. Gunnarson attended the University of Minnesota and the Minneapolis Art Institute. A print in the book *Minnesota Prints and Print Makers, 1900-1945* is attributed to him.

[23]Hannah Lokke, *Diary*, January 26, 1927. Author collection.

[24]Hannah Lokke, photograph album, 1927, and Minnesota death certificate 005447. The Poor Farm cemetery was relocated from St. Louis Park to Woodside Cemetery at Shorewood. None of the graves are marked with names.

[25]"Sheet rope victim at Glen Lake dies," *Minneapolis Tribune*, October 17, 1938.

[26]Delores Romatko Farr, interview,1990, videocassette, author's collection.

[27]*Terrace Topics*, XII, no. 7 (1945): 12. Also, Karen Krugerud, phone interview with author, April 2014.

[28]Jim Parson, "Looking back: when TB was THE dreaded U.S. disease," *Minneapolis Tribune*, April 15, 1979, sec. F.

[29]C. B. Ross and W. L. Stanbury, "Psychology of tuberculosis," *American Review of Tuberculosis*, 28 (1933): 217-228.

[30]Roger Page, "The way you see it," *Terrace Topics*, VIII, no. 11 (1941): 3.

[31]Page, "Tentative Report on 'Attitudes Study,'" *Terrace Topics*, IX, no. 7 (1942): 3, 12. Also, Roger Page, Application of the Minnesota Multiphasic Personality Inventory to Tuberculosis Patients. A thesis submitted to the graduate faculty of the University of Minnesota in partial fulfillment for the degree of doctor of philosophy, February 1947. Page retired from the University in 1988 as a psychology professor and associate dean of the College of Liberal Arts.

[32]Ernest Mariette, "Report of a year's activities of Glen Lake Sanatorium," (paper presented to the Hennepin County Medical Society and the Women's Auxiliary. Oak Terrace, MN, November 1, 1926).

[33]*Medical Staff Meeting Minutes*, April 13, May 11, 1936.

[34]*Medical Staff Meeting Minutes*, June 29, 1931.

[35]Ernest Mariette, "Report of a year's activities of Glen Lake Sanatorium."

Chapter 9

[1]Frances M. Pottenger, *Tuberculosis and How to Combat It: A Book for the Patient.* (St. Louis: C. V. Mosby Co., 1921), 209.

[2]Ernest Mariette, *Report of a Year's Activities of Glen Lake Sanatorium.* (Paper presented to the Hennepin County Medical Society and the Women's Auxiliary. November 1, 1926).

[3]Ernest Mariette, *Means of Promoting Contentment Among Patients.* (Paper presented to the Wisconsin Sanatorium Association, Muridale Sanatorium, Wawatosa, WI. June 1926).

[4]Ernest Mariette, "How Sanatorium Patients are Admitted and Their Daily Schedule," *The Modern Hospital*, XXVIII, no. 5 (1927) 3.

[5]John Stephen Wilwerding. Obituary, *Minneapolis Star Tribune*, May 5, 2012. <<http://www.legacy.com/obituaries/ startribune/obituary.aspx?n=john-stephen-wilwerding&pid=157456033>> Retrieved October 16, 2013.

[6]Ernest Mariette, *The Food Problem in a Sanatorium* (Paper presented at the 22nd meeting of the American Sanatorium Association. Indianapolis, Indiana, May 23, 1927).

[7]J. Arthur Myers, *Invited and Conquered*, 432.

[8]Charlotte Crowe, interview, 1990, videocassette, 1990, Minnetonka, MN, author collection. Also, Norma Anderson, ed., "Fred Maurer" in *San Memories* (n.p., 1990) 52.

[9]Irving Sandler, telephone conversation with author, transcript, November 1999.

[10]Mariette, *The Food Problem in a Sanatorium.*

[11]Juanita Fluery Seck, interview with author, 2013, audiocassette, Minnetonka, MN.

[12]Frederick Manfred, interview with author, 1991, videocassette, Minnetonka, MN.

[13]Wilton Lofstrand, "Our Calories," *Terrace Topics*, May 1941. 8.

[14]Norma Anderson, ed., "Lage (Lawrence) Floren" in *San Memories* (n.p., 1990) 61.

[15]Norma Anderson, ed., "Lyl Borak" in *San Memories* (n.p., 1990) 64.

[16]Norma Anderson, ed.,"Deloise Anderson Clair" in *San Memories* (n.p., 1990).

[17]*Report of the Glen Lake Sanatorium* (Oak Terrace, MN,1931) 27.

[18]Norma Anderson, ed. "Lyl Borak."

[19]Jeanette Kirby, interview, 1990, videocassette, author collection. Also, Charles Sampson, "Know your san: Agriculture, engineering, buildings, and grounds," *Terrace Topics*, 1, no. 11 (1934).

[20]John Duffy, *The Sanitarians: A History of American Public Health* (Chicago: University of Illinois Press, 1990) 198,199.

[21]Commonwealth of Pennsylvania. Department of Agriculture. "Tuberculosis of cattle and the Pennsylvania plan for its repression." *Bulletin* no. 75. <<http://www.archive.org/details/cu31924000379598>> Retrieved March 5, 2012.

[22]*Minnesota Death Index*, MNHS. Also, <<http://jenningsweb.us/cgi-bin/igmget.cgi/n=Jennings?I3557>> Retrieved March 5, 2013.

[23]"Sanitary History of Tuberculosis in Minneapolis," *Annual Reports of the Various City Officers of the City of Minneapolis, Minnesota, 1907*, 385.

[24]Myers, *Invited and Conquered*, 73.

[25]Mary Lydia Rowe and Ernest Mariette, "Occupational Therapy at Glen Lake Sanatorium," *Occupational Therapy and Rehabilitation*, III, no. 4 (1928).

[26]Myers, *Invited and Conquered*, 421.

[27]*Annual Report of the Board of Health of the Department of Health of the City of New York for the Year Ending December 31, 1908, 1*, 677.

[28]Myers, *Invited and Conquered*, 421.

[29]Norma Anderson, ed., "Anonymous" in *San Memories* (n.p., 1990) 23.

[30]Norma Anderson, ed., "Beatrice Olson" in *San Memories* (n.p., 1990) 20.

[31]Jill Young, telephone conversation with author, transcript, July 13, 2012.

[32] "Back Fence Chatter," *Terrace Topics*, IX, no. 1 (1941): 33, 47.

[33]Manuel Martinez, interview, November 3, 2001, audiocassette, Osseo, MN, author collection.

[34]*Medical Staff Meeting Minutes*, June 20, 1932.

[35]"Elks Present Altar to Glen Lake Sanatorium," *Minneapolis Star*, 1927.

[36]"Father Hays Leaves," *Terrace Topics*, September 1945.

[37]Norma Anderson, ed., "Francis Fleming" in *San Memories* (n.p., 1990) 20. Father Fleming was later a Monsignor at St. Olaf Catholic Church in Minneapolis.

[38]Glenn Gohr, "Got Any Rivers? The Story of an Inspirational Song," *Assemblies of God Heritage*. 16, no. 4 (1996-1997) 9.

[39]*Medical Staff Meeting Minutes*, April 19, 1948.

[40]"King of Swat' has Reception, Too," *Minneapolis Journal*, 1926. Undated in scrapbook, MNHS Archives.

[41]"Glen Lake catches glimpse of 'Lindy,'" *Minneapolis Tribune*, 1927. Undated clipping in scrapbook, MNHS Archives.

[42]*Medical Staff Meeting Minutes*, Dec. 21, 1942.

Chapter 10

[1]Ernest Mariette, "How Sanatorium Patients Are Admitted and Their Daily Schedule." *The Modern Hospital*, XXVIII, no. 5 (1927).

[2]J.P. Murphy, "Sanatorium Nerves," *Terrace Topics*, April 1944, p. 4.

[3]"Time capsule: 1922." *Reminisce*, December/January 2007, 19.

[4]*Medical Staff Meeting Minutes*, November 2, 1931.

[5]C.C. Sampson, "Radio," *Terrace Topics*, III, no. 6 (1936): 6.

[6]Marcella Bengtson, "Please Stand By," *Terrace Topics*, February 1936, 11.

[7]Ibid., 17.

[8]C.C. Thomas, *With Their Dying Breath* (Corydon, IN: CCThomas Writing Solutions, 2007), 108.

[9]"KNUT Staff Hard at Work," *Terrace Topics*, September 1941, p. 24.

[10]*Terrace Topics*, September 1941, 8. Also, August 1937, 26.

[11]*Terrace Topics*, December 1939.

[12]LuDean Harmson, interview.

[13]"Shriners' Party," *Terrace Topics*, II, no. 5 (1935), 15.

[14]"Easter Party at Glen Lake," *Minneapolis Star*, April 1, 1939.

[15]Norma Anderson, ed., "Deloise Anderson Clair," in *San Memories* (n.p., 1990) 16.

[16]Betty Carroll, interview, 1990, videocassette, Minnetonka, MN, author's collection.

[17]Norma Anderson, ed., "Dora Cohen," in *San Memories* (n.p.,1990) 17.

[18]*Medical Staff Meeting Minutes*, October 11, 1937.

[19]Program from the Empress, later known as the Lyceum. Lou Murray Theater papers, 1915-1931, Minnesota Historical Society.

[20]*Medical Staff Meeting Minutes*, June 18, 1928.

[21]Ernest Mariette, "How sanatorium patients are admitted and their daily schedule," 4.

[22]Norma Anderson, ed., "Phyllis Burns," in *San Memories* (n.p., 1990) 11.

[23]Don Martin, telephone conversation with author, August 15, 2002.

[24]Mary Shonka, interview, videocassette, 1990, Minnetonka, MN.

[25]Norma Anderson, ed., "Lucille Saan Douglas," in *San Memories* (n.p., 1990) 49.

[26]*Terrace Topics*, III, no. 19 (1937).

[27]Norma Anderson, ed., "Monsignor Francis J. Fleming," in *San Memories* (n.p. 1990) 20.

[28]Norma Anderson, ed., "Phyllis Burns," in *San Memories* (n.p., 1990) 11.

[29]Norma Anderson, ed., "Mary Coover Shonka," in *San Memories* (n.p. 1990) 13.

[30]*Medical Staff Meeting Minutes*, February 10, 1936.

[31]*Medical Staff Meeting Minutes*, February 9 and March 3, 1925.

[32]Judy Smykal Swedberg, phone interview, February 12, 2011, audiocassette.

[33]Don Rivers, "Visiting Made Easy," *Terrace Topics*, III, no. 11 (1936).

[34]"Visitors Find Noble Work Done at Glen Lake Sanitorium [sic]," *Excelsior-Minnetonka Record*, November 21, 1922.

[35]"Fake solicitor on job," *Minneapolis Star*, undated clipping from 1926 in Glen Lake scrapbook.

[36]"Tuberculosis and Sanitariums" in "The Friend of the People." *Minneapolis Morning Tribune*, June 9, 1921, 16.

[37]Norma Anderson, ed., "Deloise Anderson Clair," 15.

[38]Norma Anderson, ed., "Mary Coover Shonka," 14.

[39]"A Doughboy at the Cure in a Minnesota Sanatorium," *Minnesota Public Health Association Journal.* October 6, 1920, 41.

Chapter 11

[1] Jeanette Senseth. *Terrace Topics.*

[2] Jeanette Stenseth, "The Christian Memorial Children's Sanatorium," *Terrace Topics,* 6.

[3] LuDean Harmson Pontius, interview, 1990, videocassette, author's collection.

[4] Susan Oss. "Dolls and Memories," *Minneapolis StarTribune.* Also, "Trudeau Club funds," *Terrace Topics,* I, no.3, (1933) 6. Both Susan and her father were admitted to Glen Lake – she for nine months and her dad for 18 months.

[5] Stenseth, "The Christian Memorial Children's Sanatorium."

[6] Stenseth, "The Christian Memorial Children's Sanatorium."

[7] "Kiddies' Review," *Terrace Topics,* 17, August 1935.

[8] *Report of Glen Lake Sanatorium, 1934* (Oak Terrace, MN,1935) 69.

[9] *Report of Glen Lake Sanatorium, 1932-33* (Oak Terrace, MN,1934) 55.

[10] *Medical Staff Meeting Minutes,* November 17,1926.

[11] *Medical Staff Meeting Minutes,* January, 24, 1927.

[12] "Kiddies Review," *Terrace Topics,* November 1935, 18.

[13] Judy T., "Adventurers," *Terrace Topics,* November 1934.

[14] "Oletta Lunde Photo Album, 1926-1947." MNHS Archives.

[15] Norma Anderson, "Deloise Anderson Claire,"in *San Memories* (n.p., 1990) 15.

[16] Photo caption, *Minneapolis Journal.* c.1930, clipping in Glen Lake Sanatorium scrapbook, MNHS Archives.

[17] Delores Romatko Farr, interview, videocassette, 1990, author's collection.

[18] LuDean Harmson Pontius, interview.

[19] Gloria Yberra Sotello, interview, audiocassette, 2003, author's collection.

[20] Gloria Stromseth Maxson, "The Goodbye," *The Good Old Days,* Winter 1977, excerpted: Anderson, Norma, ed., "Gloria Stromseth Maxson "in *San Memories* (n.p., 1990) 76-78.

[21] Delores Romatko Farr, interview.

[22] Mel Dray, interview, videocassette, August 19, 1990, author's collection.

[23] LuDean Harmson Pontius, interview.

[24] Myers, *Invited and Conquered,* 407, 529, 682.

[25] Scott D. McGinnis, *Minnesota Visiting Nurse Agency: 100 Years of Caring for the Community.* (Minneapolis, MN: Visiting Nurse Agency, 2002), 24.

[26] *Report of the Glen Lake Sanatorium, 1932-33,* 55.

[27] Irv Hanson, "Just add water," *West Central Tribune,* Oct. 6, 1993.

[28] "Road to health is shown in boys' and girls' camps," *Northwestern Health Journal,* 10, no.8 (1925), 5.

[29] *Report of the Glen Lake Sanatorium, 1935,* 74.

[30] "Summer at Glen Lake—Swim is Daily Event," *Journal,* August 1938.

[31] "Getting Healthy Is Fun, Glen Lake Campers Find." *Minneapolis Star.* c. 1948. Undated clipping in Glen Lake Sanatorium scrapbook. MNHS Archives.

[32] "Children's Page," *Terrace Topics.* July 1942.

[33] "Getting Healthy Is Fun, Glen Lake Campers Find."

[34] "Summer at Glen Lake – Swim Is Daily Event."

[35] "The Children's Camp." *Terrace Topics,* August 1935. Also, Friends of Birch Island Woods, <http://fbiw.org>

[36]Several Glen Lake Sanatorium annual reports from the 1930s mention Mrs. George Chase Christian's visits to the summer camp and the Children's Building.
[37]*Report of the Glen Lake Sanatorium, 1931,* 25.
[38]Earl Leaf, E-mail to author, January 16, 2013.

Chapter 12
[1]"A Letter to a new patient," *Terrace Topics,* November 1942, 13.
[2]Judy Smykal Swedberg, phone interview with author, February 12, 2011, author collection.
[3]In May 1950 the *Journal of the American Medical Association* published a paper saying that lung cancer occurred almost exclusively in smokers. <<http://www.nytimes.com/1988/06/17/us/smoking-and-cancer-what-cigarette-concerns-really-knew.html?pagewanted=all&src=pm>>
[4]*Terrace Topics,* I, no.2, (1933).
[5]*Medical Staff Meeting Minutes,* Oct. 12, 1925.
[6]*Medical Staff Meeting Minutes,* Jan 26, 1931; August 10, 1931; May 20, 1929.
[7]*General laws of Minnesota for 1913.* Chapter 434 – S.F. No. 201, Section 3.
[8]Minnesota Department of Health, *Minnesota's Health,* V, no. 6, (1951) 3.
[9]*Medical Staff Meeting Minutes,* March 9, 1925.
[10]*Medical Staff Meeting Minutes,* March 19, 1928.
[11]*Medical Staff Meeting Minutes,* May 20, 1929; October 14, 1929; September 29, 1930, July 26, 1943.
[12]*Medical Staff Meeting Minutes,* February 1, 1927.
[13]*Handbook for Patients at Glen Lake Sanatorium,* Oak Terrace, MN.
[14]Norma Anderson, ed., "Pernilla Lembke," in *San Memories* (n.p., 1990) 69.
[15]Carol Anderson, interview by author, March 2010, audiocassette. Author collection.
[16]Catherine Hanitch, telephone interview with Norma Anderson, n.d.
[17]*Medical Staff Meeting Minutes,* December 17, 1928; January 7 and January 14, 1929.
[18]*Medical Staff Meeting Minutes,* August 30, 1926, and January 4, 1927.
[19]*Report of Glen Lake Sanatorium, 1935.* Oak Terrace, MN.
[20]Sheila Rothman, *Living in the Shadow of Death,* (New York: Basic Books, 1994), 236.
[21]*Medical Staff Meeting Minutes,* April 1, 1929.
[22]"The Doghouse," *Terrace Topics,* January 1938.
[23]Norma Anderson, ed., "Dora Cohen," 63.
[24]Norma Anderson, ed., "Howard and Lois Johnson," 66.
[25]Norma Anderson, ed., "Phyllis Burns," 11.
[26]Gloria Belitz Alstrup, interview, August 19, 1990, videocassette, Minnetonka, MN.
[27]Frederick Manfred, interview, August 19, 1990, videocassette, Minnetonka, MN.
[28]*Transactions of the Minnesota State Medical Association* (St. Paul: Northwestern Lancet, 1897) 69.
[29]Evelyn Roland Wolter, online obituary reprinted with permission from *The Hudson Star-Observer,* March 1, 2002. Retrieved May 1, 2014, from <<http://archiver.rootsweb.ancestry.com/th/read/WISTCROI/2002.>>

[30]Victor Funk, MD, interview, 1990, videocassette, Minnetonka, MN. Mrs. Funk lived to be eighty-six without any reactivation of TB.
[31]*Medical Staff Meeting Minutes*, November 25, 1928.
[32]Helen Mary Vavra and Albert James Kranz, *The Dvoraks of Minnetonka Township Minnesota* (Minneapolis: Albert Kranz, 1988).
[33]<<http://archiver.rootsweb.ancestry.com/th/read/WIDOUGLA/2008-11/1227399534>> retrieved November 17, 2013. Also, 1930 U. S. Census.
[34]Oberg, Adele Boquist, letter, August 1942. She was discharged in 1928.
[35]*Medical Staff Meeting Minutes*, July 1 and July 8, 1929.
[36]Norma Anderson, ed., "Deloise Anderson Clair," 18.
[37]Mary Shonka, interview, 1990, videocassette. Author collection.
[38]*Medical Staff Meeting Minutes*, November 23, 1942.
[39]Edwin Black, Remarks relating to my spontaneous and unrehearsed testimony before the house judiciary committee's subcommittee on the constitution on the historical question of eugenics and racism. Washington, D.C., Dec. 6, 2011. Retrieved October 6, 2012. <<http://judiciary.house.gov/hearings.pdf/black12062011.pdf>>
[40]Allen K. Krause, quoted in J. Arthur Myers, *Invited and Conquered*, 480.
[41]William Darity, Jr., ed., *Race, Radicalism, and Reform*; selected papers, Abram L. Harris. (New Brunswick, NJ: Transaction Publishers, 1989) 69.
[42]Hennepin County Tuberculosis Association, *Twenty-five years of fighting tuberculosis in Minneapolis and Hennepin County, 1903-1928* (Minneapolis: HCTA, 1928) 26, 29.
[43]*Medical Staff Meeting Minutes*, March 21, 1927.
[44]*Medical Staff Meeting Minutes*, June 6, 1927.
[45]"Ah-gwah-ching 'E' or Eagle Building," *Cass County Clippings*, April 1, 2009: 1, 3.
[46]Ray Earley, phone interview with author, February 6, 2014.
[47]*Terrace Topics*, November 1935, 18.
[48]"Fond Flashback, 1928," *Reminisce*, July/August 2002, 19.
[49]Charlotte Keyes, *Glen Lake Sanatorium: A Report to Administration* (n.p. April 12, 1947)
[50]Minnesota Medical Association, *Minnesota Medicine*, 9, no. 3 (1926) 116-119.

Chapter 13

[1]*Report of Glen Lake Sanatorium, 1931*, Oak Terrace, MN: Glen Lake Sanatorium Vocational School (1932), 8.
[2]Raymond Koch, "Politics and Relief in Minneapolis during the 1930s," *Minnesota History*, 41, no. 4, (1968), 153.
[3]*Report of Glen Lake Sanatorium, 1932-1933*, (1934), 6.
[4]*Report of Glen Lake Sanatorium, 1934*, (1935), 10.
[5]*Report of Glen Lake Sanatorium, 1932-1933*, 15.
[6]*Medical Staff Meeting Minutes*, Oct 10, 1932.
[7]*Medical Staff Meeting Minutes*, May 8, 1933.
[8]*Medical Staff Meeting Minutes*, July 21 1930.
[9]*Report of Glen Lake Sanatorium, 1932-1933*, 41. Also, Mary Coover Shonka and Margaret Jarrett, interviews, videocassette, Aug. 19, 1990, Minnetonka, MN.

[10]*Report of Glen Lake Sanatorium, 1935*, 10.

[11]Charles K. Petter, "An attachment for Hawley Fracture Table," *Journal of Bone and Joint Surgery*, XVI, no.1 (1934), 211; Charles K. Petter, "Handy bone grasping forceps," *Journal of Bone and Joint Surgery*, XVIII, no.4 (1936), 1084.

[12]*Report of Glen Lake Sanatorium, 1932-1933*, 21.

[13]*Report of Glen Lake Sanatorium, 1932-1933*, 23.

[14]*Report of Glen Lake Sanatorium, 1932-1933*, 19-21.

[15]"Winnipeg M.D. Lauds Glen Lake," *Terrace Topics*, III, no. 5 (1936), 13.

[16]*Terrace Topics*, I, no.5 (1934), 8.

[17]*Terrace Topics*. Various issues. The regionally popular Schmidt beer was brewed in St. Paul. Glueks brewery in Minneapolis was the first in the state. Jordan was brewed in and named after a city about 25 miles southwest of the sanatorium.

[18]Norma Anderson, ed., "Wayne Engstrom," in *San Memories* (n.p., 1990), 9.

[19]Raymond Koch, 154,157.

[20]Patient Record of Admissions. MNHS archives. Also, Betty Carroll, interview, videocassette, 1990, Minnetonka, MN.

[21]Patient Record of Admissions. MNHS archives.

[22]Norma Anderson, ed., "Betty Carroll," 55; and *Medical Staff Meeting Minutes*, June 30, 1952.

[23]Norma Anderson, ed., "Phyllis Burns," 12.

[24]*Medical Staff Meeting Minutes*, September 18 , 1933 and October 17, 1938.

[25]Frank L. Jennings and Ernest S. Mariette, "A Biometric study of pregnancy and tuberculosis," *The American Review of Tuberculosis*, XXV, no. 6 (1932), 673-694. Also, *Medical Staff Meeting Minutes*, Sept 19, 1932.

[26]*Medical Staff Meeting Minutes*, Nov 27, 1933.

[27]J. Arthur Myers, "Entrance, Rise, and Fall of Tuberculosis in Minnesota," *Minnesota Medicine*, 60, no. 9 (1977), 681.

[28]Frank L. Jennings, "Tuberculosis infection and morbidity among medical students and physicians." *Minnesota Medicine*. February 1938, v. 21, p 102-105. MNHS archives.

[29]Myers, "Entrance, rise, and Fall of Tuberculosis in Minnesota," 681.

[30]*Medical Staff Meeting Minutes*, May 25 1925, March 26 1928.

[31]*Medical Staff Meeting Minutes*, Dec. 27 1937.

[32]*Medical Staff Meeting Minutes*, Sept 27 1937.

Chapter 14

[1]*Medical Staff Meeting Minutes*, April 24, 1939. The meat handler lived to be 82.

[2]<<http://www.demographicchartbook.com>> The 1930 census did not ask for educational level.

[3]Myers, *Invited and Conquered*, 424-425.

[4]"Graduates Gang Up on Us," *Terrace Topics*, III, no. 20, (1937), 12.

[5]*50 years of Fighting Tuberculosis in Hennepin County, 1903-1953*, Minneapolis: Hennepin County Tuberculosis Association.

[6]*Report of Glen Lake Sanatorium, 1931* (Oak Terrace, MN: Glen Lake Sanatorium Vocational School, 1932): 8.

[7]"Clarence Bowers Marks Up Brilliant Records, Doing Greater Part of His Work at Sanatorium – to Leave Soon," *Minneapolis Journal*, June 15, 1934.

[8]Norma Anderson, ed., "Beatrice Olson," in *San Memories* (n.p., 1990) 21.

[9]Norma Anderson, ed., "Mary Shonka," 14.

[10]Holland Hudson, "Young Married Women Patients: Rehabilitation Lacking for This Group in Which Percentage of Relapses is High," *Terrace Topics*, XII, no.3 (1944) 3, 4. Reprint of a National Tuberculosis Association bulletin.

[11]*Report of Glen Lake Sanatorium, 1934*, 66, 67.

[12]"About the Print Shop," *Terrace Topics*, III, no. 19 (1937) 7.

[13]*Terrace Topics*, 1, no. 9 (1934) 5.

[14]"Dishing Out the Dirt," *Terrace Topics*, III, no. 6 (1936) 16.

[15]Gloria Stromseth Maxson, Kennings, (Boston: Branden Press, 1974): 39. Maxson wrote in five-line cinquain verse-form, a very strict structure also used by American poet Adelaide Crapsey who was a patient at Saranac Lake in 1913.

[16]Don Rivers, "A Gentleman in Bed: The Episode of The Lady in Blue," *Terrace Topics*, II, no.12, (1935) 6, 12.

[17]"Alumni News," *Terrace Topics*, III, no. 14 (1936) 14.

[18]*Report of Glen Lake Sanatorium, 1932-1933*, 10.

[19]Yvonne DeBere Alexander, interview, videocassette, August 19, 1990, Minnetonka, MN.

[20]Delores Romatko Farr, interview, videocassette, August 19, 1990, Minnetonka, MN.

[21]*Terrace Topic*, III, no. 9, (1936), 11. Also, Margaret McConaughey Jarrett, interview, August 19, 1990, videocassette.

[22]D'Antonio, Patricia, et al. *Nurses' Work: Issues across Time and Place*. (New York: Springer Publishing, 2007): 181.

[23]Norma Anderson, ed. "Dora Cohen," 62.

[24]Arlene Geuder Graupmann, interview, videocassette, August 19, 1990, Minnetonka, MN.

[25]Ruth Altland, e-mail to author, April 25, 2002.

[26]"Honor Student," *Terrace Topics*, VI, no. 10 (1939): 28. Also http://www.joan-styve.net/Family/WebDocuments/Blog-PernillaLembke.pdf.

[27]"For Women Only," *Terrace Topics*, VIII, no. 7, (1941).

[28]Lael Withrow, "Working at Glen Lake was her 'compensation' for TB," *Minneapolis Sunday Tribune*, Jan. 21, 1962.

[29]Myers, J. Arthur. *Invited and Conquered*, 183.

[30]"Sarahurst, the House the Christmas Seals Keep," *Terrace Topics*, IV (1937).

[31]"Restored," *Terrace Topics*, II, no.3, (1939).

[32]"Visitor will study tuberculosis work," *Minneapolis Star-Journal*, Sep 9, 1939.

[33]"Baseball Thrills," *Terrace Topics*, August. 1935. P. 14.

[34]Sandler, Irving, phone interview with author, November 1999.

[35]*Report of Glen Lake Sanatorium, 1936*, p. 11.

[36]"Glen Lake Patients Hear Symphony Orchestra in Concert," *Minneapolis Journal*, November 27, 1935.

[37]"Entertainment," *Terrace Topics*, VI, no. 2 (1938), 17.

[38]"The Stage Scenery." *Terrace Topics*. May 1937. Charles Wells was on the faculty of the Minneapolis School of Art until 1931 and did ornamental work on several local buildings. After an absence from Minnesota, he taught in Minneapolis under the Federal Art Project until retirement in 1941. Source: Charles S. Wells manuscript collection, Minnesota Historical Society. Stanley Waldo moved to California and did work for Disney. Source: Clement B. Haupers oral history. December 9, 1977. Minnesota Historical Society.

[39]"Entertainers," *Terrace Topics*, II, no. 8 (1935), 17.

[40]"Notes on the Staff," *Terrace Topics*, III, no. 14, (1936) 4. Also, Report of Glen Lake Sanatorium, 1936, 98.

[41]Myers, *Invited and Conquered*, 147. Also, Mary Shonka, interview.

[42]*Consumers Guide*, Catalogue No. 110, (Chicago: Sears, Roebuck and Co., 1990 reprint).

[43]"Cure Taking in Java," *Terrace Topics*, VI, no. 8 (1939) 7.

[44]C--, M--, "Portrait of a pacifist," *Terrace Topics*, III, 20 (1937) 13. Scherling had been the superintendent of the Talmud Torah, Mikro Kodesh congregation in Minneapolis. Telz is the Yiddish name for Telsiai.

[45]"Back Fence Chatter, Second East," T*errace Topics*, VI, no. 10 (1939), 18.

Chapter 15

[1]Maryanna Shorba, Diary.

[2]"Telling the Children. Skulls to Cartoons," National Tuberculosis Association. Goodbye Mr. Germ. Film. Directed by Edgar Ulmer (1940). <https://www.you-tube.com/watch?v=xuEMRKY5R1c>. Retrieved August 17, 2014.

[3]*Medical Staff Meeting Minutes*, August 12, 1940, February 9, 1942.

[4]Norma Anderson, ed., "Myrtle Johnson," in *San Memories* (n.p., 1990), 25-26.

[5]Theresa Ledermann Lanners, interview with author, August 23, 2000, audiocassette.

[6]Al Greene, "The Song of the Buy-o," *Terrace Topics*, VIII, no. 10, (1941).

[7]*Medical Staff Meeting Minutes,* November 11, 1940.

[8]Worthy Turner, "A Democratic Quirk" *Terrace Topics*, VIII, no. 12 (1941), 4.

[9]Wilton Lofstrand, "Racial Prejudice," *Terrace Topics*, IX, no. 1(1941), 29.

[10]*Medical Staff Meeting Minutes*, July 21, 1947.

[11]Feike Feikema, "Black cat murder," *Terrace Topics*, IX, no. 3 (1941) 5.

[12]Frederick Manfred, interview, videocassette, August 19, 1990. Minnetonka, MN. That sentiment was also expressed by Eugene O'Neill, who incorporated his tuberculosis experience into his plays, *Long Day's Journey into Night and The Straw*.

[13]Feike Feikema, "Hubert the Tuber Complains," *Terrace Topics*, VIII, no. 5 (1941)16. Also appears in April 1941 in "Hubert Discusses Human Dignity," 11, and "Hubert the Tuber Encourages Revolt" in June 1941, 6.

[14]*Medical Staff Meeting Minutes*, December 28, 1942, 205

[15]Jean S. Mason, "The Discourse of Disease: 'Patient Writes' at the 'University of Tuberculosis.'" <<http://web.english.ufl.edu/pnm/mason.html.>> Retrieved September 17, 2012.

[16]*Medical Staff Meeting Minutes*, December 22, 1941 and January 18, 1943.

[17]Norma Anderson, ed., "Victor Funk," 6.

[18]Norma Anderson, ed., "Norman Distad," 49.

[19]"Nurses' Aides Put in Busy Evening," *Minnetonka Record*, October 20, 1942.

[20]Norma Anderson, ed., "Virginia Schwarting," 57. Also, article in Olletta Lunde scrapbook in MNHS Archives.

[21]*Medical Staff Meeting Minutes*, March 16, 1942.

[22]"Sanatorium Facts," *Terrace Topics*, IX, no. 6 (1942), 7.

[23]"Sugar and Bullets," *Terrace Topics*, X (1943).

[24]"Rationing and How It Affects Glen Lake Sanatorium" *Terrace Topics*, X (1943). Also, "Glen Lake head dietician to retire after 25 years," *Minneapolis Star Journal*, November 6, 1941.

[25]"Use it Up," *Terrace Topics*, XII (1945).

[26]*Medical Staff Meeting Minutes*, December 20, 1943.

[27]"Children's Page" *Terrace Topics*, May 1943.

[28]*Terrace Topics*, June 1944.

[29]"Recent Changes in Nursing Care in the Sanatorium," *Terrace Topics*, July 1943.

[30]*Medical Staff Meeting Minutes*, September 14 and September 23, 1942.

[31]*Report of Glen Lake Sanatorium, 1942-43*, 61.

[32]Barbara Meyer Bistodeau, "The Cadet Nurse Corps," April 4, 2007, retrieved from <<http:www.camdennews.org>>

[33]Buelah Baxter, interview, videocassette, August 19, 1990. Also, Norma Anderson, ed., "Phyllis Burns,"10. Also, Margaret Anderson, interview, videocassette, 1990, Minnetonka, MN

[34]"Cadet Nurse Ruled Employee of University," *Minneapolis Star*, December 10, 1949.

[35]"Student Nurses at Glen Lake Sanatorium," *Terrace Topics*, August 1945.

[36]Charlotte Crowe, interview, 1990, videocassette, Minnetonka, MN.

[37]*Report of Glen Lake Sanatorium*, 61.

[38]"Glen Lake Gets 6 Japs," *Minneapolis Star Tribune*, May 17, 1943. Also, "San Staff is Short Nurses and Doctors," *Hennepin County Review*, May 27, 1943.

[39]"Nurses and Employees' News," *Terrace Topics*, May 1943.

[40]John Hobuya Tsuchida, *Reflections: Memoirs of Japanese American Women in Minnesota* (Pacific Asia Press, 1995) 204.

[41]Tom Hara, interview with author, October 2012.

[42]*Terrace Topics*, X, no. 3 (1942).

[43]*Medical Staff Meeting Minutes*, November 22, 1943.

[44]*Medical Staff Meeting Minutes*, January 19, 1925; November 22, 1937.

[45]*Medical Staff Meeting Minutes*, April 6, 1942.

[46]*Report of Glen Lake Sanatorium 1942-43*, 13.

Chapter 16

[1]"Board Wrangles Over Sister Kenny Clinic," *Minneapolis Tribune*, August 1942.

[2]"Fight Resumed on Tuberculosis Authority in City," *Minneapolis Daily Times*, March 10, 1942. Also, Leonard Wilson, "Variety Heart Hospital and Glen Lake" *Medical Revolution and Star Journal*, November 18, 1943.

[3]"Child Enemy [incomplete headline]," *Minneapolis Star-Journal*, November 18, 1943.

[4]"Tuberculosis Deaths Rise" *Minneapolis Star-Journal*, November 12, 1944.

[5]"Glen Lake Tavern Refused License," *Minneapolis Star-Journal*, June 29, 1942.

[6]"Official Calls Charges against Sanatorium Unfair Half-Truths," September 17, 1944. Also, "Jury Foreman Answers Critic," *Minneapolis Star-Journal*, October 1, 1944.

[7]"Ask Committee on Incorrigible Patients Problem," *Minneapolis Daily Times*, September 21, 1945.

[8]"Employees' News," *Terrace Topics*, June 1945.

[9]*Medical Staff Meeting Minutes*, January 31, 1944.

[10]Albert Q. Maisel, "The Veteran betrayed," *Reader's Digest*, April 1945, 45-50.

[11]"Veterans Hospital Heads Attack Magazine Charges," *Minneapolis Star-Journal*, April 11, 1945.

[12]Albert Q. Maisel, "General Bradley Cleans up the Veterans' Hospitals." *Reader's Digest*, December 1945, 85-88.

[13]"Vets Urge T.B. Men be Kept at Snelling," *St. Paul Pioneer Press*, August 12, 1945.

[14]*Medical Staff Meeting Minutes*, February 3, 1947. Also, J. Arthur Myers, *Invited and Conquered*, 475.

[15]Thomas Saylor, interview with Harold Kurvers, March 18, 2002. Retrieved November 14, 2004. <<http://www.lindavdahl.com/Bio%20Pages/H.Kurvers/H.Kurvers.bio.htm>>.

[16]"Hopkins Legionnaires initiated members at Glen Lake sanatorium," *Hennepin County Review*, October 31, 1947.

[17]*Medical Staff Meeting Minutes*, November 15 and December 20, 1948.

[18]Jim Parsons, "Looking back: When TB was THE Dreaded U.S. Disease," *Minneapolis Tribune*, Sec. F.

[19]Online sources including Ancestry.com, MNHS.org, and discovernikkei.org.

[20]forteachers/upload/ShishinoH.pdf>>.

[21]Shih Hao Tsai, interview with author, 1990, videocassette.

[22]Jeff Yue, interview with author, 2016, audiocassette.

[23]*Head Nurses Meetings*, Glen Lake Sanatorium, September 23, 1941. MNHS Archives.

[24]"Two Mayo Doctors Protest Article on Their TB Cure," *Minneapolis Morning Tribune*, August 11, 1944.

[25]*Medical Staff Meeting Minutes*, June 1941 and April 1944.

[26]Frank Ryan, *Tuberculosis: The Greatest Story Never Told* (England: Swift Publishers, 1992): 229.

[27]David Eugene Williams, "I Remember. . . Patsy's Cure." Retrieved February 24, 2014. <<http://www-archive.thoracic.org/sections/about-ats/centennial/vignettes/articles/ vignette4.html>>

[28]"Mayo Doctor Cites Uses of Streptomycin Drug," *Minneapolis Star*, June 17, 1947.

[29]Norma Anderson, ed., "Dora Cohen," 63.

[30]*Medical Staff Meeting Minutes*, December 24, 1945.

[31]Norma Anderson, ed., "Fred Maurer," 53.

[32]Norma Anderson, ed., "Deloise Anderson Clair," 16.

[33]*Medical Staff Meeting Minutes*, April 7 and July 28, 1947.

[34]"5 Wait Yule in Hospital." *Minneapolis Star*, December 10, 1947.

[35]"Girl Owes Life to Streptomycin: Drug Licks 100% Fatal Disease." Undated clipping in Glen Lake Sanatorium Scrapbook. M---- June or July 1948 or 49

[36]Victor Cohn, "Drug Heads off 'Sure Death' TB," *Minneapolis Sunday Tribune*, Undated clipping in Glen Lake Sanatorium Scrapbook, and "Rare Drug Saves Jimmy's Life," *Minneapolis Labor Review*, October 2, 1947.

[37]Norma Anderson, ed., "Phyllis Munson Burns," 12.

[38]*Medical Staff Meeting Minutes*, October 18, 1948.

[39]Frank Ryan, The Forgotten Plague, (Boston: Little, Brown, & Company, 1993): 331.

[40]Norma Anderson, ed., "Wayne Engstrom,"9. Also, "Robert Engstrom," 9, and "Nancy Rootes," 7.

[41]"Glen Lake San Observes Anniversary: Synonym of Rest, Recuperation 45 Years," *Hennepin County Review*, May 4, 1961.

[42]Victor Funk, interview, 1990, videocassette.

[43]"New Public Health Center Opens," *Terrace Topics*, September 1945.

[44]"Ask Heart Clinic be Moved from Kenny Institute," *Minneapolis Star Journal*, October 19, 1945.

Chapter 17

[1]"Tuberculosis End Forecast by 1966," *Minneapolis Journal*, November 12, 1946. Myers' statement had been published in a pamphlet titled, "Public Health Reports."

[2]Milt Hakel, "Noted Sanatorium Head Led Fight to Whip TB," *Hennepin County Review*, September 22, 1949.

[3]"Sanatorium Deficit Seen," *Minneapolis Star-Journal*, December 12, 1946.

[4]"Sanatorium Head Hits Back at 'U' Professor," *Minneapolis Daily Times*, November 12, 1946.

[5]"Sanatorium '47 Outlook Dark for Lack of Funds," *The Spectator*, January 1, 1947.

[6]"What Do You Think?" *Minneapolis Times*, February 11, 1947. Also, "Glen Lake Fund Pleas Indorsed [sic]," *Minneapolis Sunday Tribune*, March 16, 1947.

[7]"Glen Lake Starts to Show Political Complications," *The Spectator*, February 7, 1947. Also, "City Payroll Tax Pushed," *Minneapolis Tribune*, March 22, 1947.

[8]"W.N. Lundahl has resigned at Glen Lake," *Hennepin County Review*, October 2, 1947.

[9]"Would Take Power from Commission," *The Spectator*, February 7, 1947.

[10]Session Laws, State of Minnesota, 1947, Chapter 370 and 598.

[11]"Glen Lake to Take 'Drastic Action' to Gain More Room," *Minneapolis Morning Tribune*, April 29, 1947. Also, "Glen Lake to Lose Revenues in Patient Shift," *Minneapolis Star*, November 11, 1947. Also, "Ruling Asked on Glen Lake Vet Ouster," *Minneapolis Star*, November 8, 1947.

[12]"More Glen Lake Beds," n.p., December 6, 1947. Clipping illegible.

[13]Elizabeth Emerson, *Public Health Is People: A History of the Minnesota Department of Health, 1949-1999* (St. Paul), 46.

[14]"19 at Glen Lake to Be Evicted," *Minneapolis Sunday Tribune*, November 2, 1947.

[15]"Sanatorium '47 Outlook Dark for Lack of Funds." Undated clipping in Glen Lake Sanatorium Scrapbook. MNHS Archives.

[16]"First of DPs to Join Glen Lake Staff in January," newspaper unknown. December 30, 1948.

[17]Judy Smykal Swedberg, phone conversation with author, February 12, 2011, audiocassette.

[18]"DP Romance: Diamond Ring Lights Way to Altar for Pair," *Minneapolis Star*, March 10, 1949.

[19]"Latvian DP Studies at San for MD Exams," *Hennepin County Review*, November 3, 1949.

[20]"Classical Hour," *Terrace Topics*, January 1942.

[21]Bill Carlson, "Delores Autey Speeds to Health," *Minneapolis Star-Journal*, November 5, 1946. Delores left Glen Lake, married, and died in 2002.

[22]Virgil Israelson, interview with author, October 13, 2014, audiocassette.

[23]Photo with caption, *Minneapolis Star-Journal*, August 29, 1946.

[24]Art Hager, "Just Ask the Men," *Minneapolis Morning Tribune*, March 6, 1947, p. 14.

[25]"'Wheelchair Post Office' Really Rollin'," *Minneapolis Star Journal*, December 19, 1945.

[26]"After Glen Lake Blast," *Minneapolis Star-Journal*, September 19, 1946.

[27]Minnesota State Fair History. Retrieved August 2, 2016. <<http://www.mnstatefair.org/pdf/media/MSF_History.pdf>

[28]"Glen Lake Patients Win Prizes," *Minneapolis Sunday Tribune*, August 1947. Also, "Glen Lake Patients Win Fair Titles," unknown paper, August 30, 1948.

[29]"Drinking Patients are a Problem at Sanitarium [sic]," *The Mail of Minneapolis*. 2, no. 20, (1948).

[30]*Medical Staff Meeting Minutes*, April 19, 1948.

[31]*Medical Staff Meeting Minutes*, May 23 and June 27, 1949.

[32]"County has Sanatorium Fund Deficit," *Minneapolis Star*, July 27, 1949, 28.

[33]"Glen Lake Sanatorium 'In the Black'," *Minneapolis Star*, August 12, 1949.

[34]Grace Mariette Norris, interview by author, 2004, audiocassette, Minnetonka, MN.

[35]"Dr. Ernest Sidney Mariette Retires," *Oak Leaves*, II, no. 4 (1949).

[36]*Terrace Topics*, XVIII, (1950) 8,10.

[37]Elizabeth Emerson, *Public Health Is People*, 46.

Chapter 18

[1]Walter Johnson, "TB patient sees baby first time," *Minneapolis Star*, January 2, 1950.

[2]*Terrace Topics*, XVIII, no. 4 (1950).

[3]*Medical Staff Meeting Minutes*, January 30, 1950.

[4]Myers, JA "Entrance, Rise, and Fall of Tuberculosis in Minnesota."

[5]*Medical Staff Meeting Minutes*, October 30, 1950.

[6]*Medical Staff Meeting Minutes*, September 8, 1950.

[7]Minnesota Board of Health, *Minutes*, January 25, 1951, 54-56.

[8]*Medical Staff Meeting Minutes*, February 13, 1950.

[9]September 15, 1952, background information from 117.g.8.7b, MNHS

[10]*Medical Staff Meeting Minutes*, September 8, 1952

[11]"Wedding Bells," *Minneapolis Star*, November 28, 1952.

[12]Frances Lange, interview with author, July 9, 2010, audiocassette.

[13]MNHS, 109.K.6.10F.Box 1. Folder : Correspondence with other Hosp. re. GLS procedures, 1954-1959.

[14]Gordon Snider, "Tuberculosis Then and Now: A Personal Perspective on the Last 50 Years," *Annals of Internal Medicine*. 126, no. 3, (1997) 237-243.

[15]Carol Anderson, interview with author, 2010, audiocassette.

[16]Martin Kawano, from unpublished manuscript sent to author in 1990. Later edited by Paul W. Miller and published as *The Cloud and the Light* by Cross Cultural Publications, 1997.

[17]Manuel Martinez, interview with author, November 3, 2001, audiocassette.

[18]Norma Anderson, ed., "Howard Johnson," 66.

[19]Myers, J. Arthur, "Entrance, Rise, and Fall of Tuberculosis in Minnesota."

[20]Elizabeth Emerson, *Public Health Is People*, 53.

[21]Minnesota Tuberculosis Facilities Commission, Tuberculosis Control in Minnesota, January 1955, 16.

[22]Glen Lake statistics from box 109.K.6.10.F at the Minnesota Historical Society Archives.

[23]"Let's Look at the Record – Progress in Controlling TB" *Everybody's Health*. June, July, August 1956. 20

[24]*Detroit Lakes Tribune*, April 12, 1951, 6.

[25]"Legal Opinion Expressed in Closing of Fair Oaks Lodge," *Wadena Pioneer Journal*, 74, no. 28 (1951) 1.

[26]*Citizens League Report*, No. 66, Glen Lake Sanatorium, Operational Review. February 1957. 4, 5, 6. The Citizens League was established in 1952.

[27]"Glen Lake 'San' Observes Anniversary: Synonym of Rest, Recuperation 45 Years," *Hennepin County Review*, May 4, 1961.

[28]*Minneapolis Star*, October 7, 1958.

[29]Daniel J. Hafrey, "State Examiner Charges Law Violations and Waste at Glen Lake Sanatorium," *Minneapolis Morning Tribune*, February 25, 1959, 1,6,16.

[30]Jacqueline Adams, "Grand Jury Assails Ex-Glen Lake Board, *Minneapolis Morning Tribune*, June 11, 1959, 1,5.

[31]"New Broom at Glen Lake," *Minneapolis Morning Tribune*, September 14, 1959, P.6.

[32]Al Woodruff, "Nursing Home Role Urged for Glen Lake," *Minneapolis Star*, January 6, 1960, Sec. A.

[33]Dorothy Smith, "Glen Lake's 'New Broom' Criticized," *Minneapolis Morning Tribune*, Sept. 26, 1959, 4.

[34]Al Woodruff, "Nursing Home Role Urged For Glen Lake." Undated clipping in Glen Lake Sanatorium Scrapbook. MNHS Archives.

[35]Irving Juster, "Glen Lake Nursing Home," *The Minneapolis Star*, May 9, 1960.

[36]William Goldberg, "Glen Lake Nursing Home," *The Minneapolis Star*, sec. A, June 23, 1960.

[37]"Group Urges Glen Lake to Reject Change," *Minneapolis Sunday Tribune*, January 10, 1960.

Chapter 19

[1]"Plan would convert Glen Lake San to home for elderly mental patients," *Hennepin County Review*, January 12, 1961, 6.

[2]Maury Treberg, interview with Colleen Spadaccini, videocassette, 1990.

[3]Karla Wennerstrom, Eden Prairie News, Wednesday, May 10, 2006. Retrieved February 9, 2015 from <<http://fbiw.net/old_site/Archive/EdenWoodTLC.htm>>

[4]A Little History. Retrieved April 30, 2014 from <<http://www.conferenceandretreat.org/history>>.

[5]Laws 1961 c618. Bill S.F. No. 175 chapter 52 of extra session, 1961, HF no 1151, chapter 118 1961.

[6]*Glen Lake Sanatorium*, Published records and reports, Minnesota State Archives.

[7]Sam Newlund, "County TB Sanatorium to Get New Look as State Nursing Home," *Minneapolis Sunday Tribune*, December 17, 1961, 4.

[8]Judy Scholer, Interview, August 19, 1990, videocassette.

[9]Margaret Klosterman Anderson, interview, 1990, videocassette.

[10]Charlotte Crowe, interview, 1990, videocassette.

[11]Betty Carroll, interview, 1990, videocassette.

[12]Paulette Anderson, interview, 1990, videocassette.

[13]"Life and Times are Good at Oak Terrace," *Minnetonka Sun Sailor*, July 4, 1979, sec. A.

[14]Jarvis Hauger, Interview, August 19, 1990.

[15]Norma Anderson, ed., "Dora Cohen," in *San Memories* (n.p., 1990) 63.

[16]Ramona Ebert Pockrandt, interview, 1990, videocassette.

[17]Norma Anderson, interview, 1990, videocassette.

[18]Sam Newlund, "County TB Sanatorium to Get New Look as State Nursing Home."

[19]Raymond Sotelo, interview with author, audiocassette.

[20]*Glen Lake Sanatorium*, Published records and reports, Minnesota State Archives.

[21]Catherine Johnson, interview with Colleen Spadaccini, 1990, videocassette.

[22]Maury Treberg, interview.

[23]Letter to Mr. Alfon Hanson from Lilja A. Syder, R.N. and Polk County Public Health nurse, April 6, 1967.

[24]Catherine Johnson, interview.

[25]Neil Hering, interview, 1990, videocassette.

[26]Ibid.

[27]Don Jones, interview, 1990, videocassette.

[28]Maury Treberg, interview.

[29]Margaret Kienzle, interview,1990, videocassette. The quilts were later donated to the Minnesota Historical Society and the Hennepin County Historical Society.

[30]Myrtle Murk, interview, August 19, 1990, videocassette.

[31]"Glen Lake Sanatorium Slated for Demolition." Preservation Matters, *Preservation Alliance of Minnesota*, January 1993, 3.

Chapter 20

[1] Irwin W. Sherman, *Twelve Diseases that Changed the World* (Washington, D.C.: ASM Press, 2007): 121.

[2] John F. Briggs and J. Arthur Myers, "Tuberculosis Eradication Plan of Minnesota Medical Association," *Diseases of the Chest* 42 (1962): 279.

[3] "Question Box," *Terrace Topics*, January 1938.

[4] Leslie Maitland, "The Design of Tuberculosis Sanatoria in Late Nineteenth Century Canada, *Bulletin*, 14, no.1 (1989):13.

[5] Henry M. Bracken, "State Aid for Sanatoria for the Tuberculous." Paper presented at the Mississippi Valley Conference on Tuberculosis. Louisville, KY, Oct. 5, 1916.

[6] "Let's Look at the Record – Progress in Controlling TB," *Everybody's Health* (June, July, August, 1956): 20.

[7] Masahiti (Martin) Kawano, Statistical Study of Pulmonary Resection Cases at Glen Lake Sanatorium, 1953. Unpublished report.

[8] Herbert Lampson, "A Study on the Spread of Tuberculosis in Families," *Bulletin of the University of Minnesota*, 1913.

[9] Karen Krugerud, telephone conversation with author, April 17, 2014.

[10] Norma Anderson, interview, video tape.

[11] *Report of Glen Lake Sanatorium, 1937*. Sanatorium Commission of Hennepin County. (Oak Terrace, MN: Glen Lake Sanatorium Vocational School) 49-54.

[12] Charles Phillips Emerson, *Essentials of Medicine*, 13th edition, 1939, Philadelphia: J. B. Lippincott Company.679.

[13] Juanita Fleury Seck, interview by author. Audiocassette, March 2012. Author collection.

[14] Huseboe, Arthur R. and Nancy Owen Nelson, eds. *The Selected Letters of Frederick Manfred, 1932-1954*. (Lincoln: University of Nebraska Press, 1989): 122, 125.

[15] Norma Anderson, ed., *San Memories*, 1990.

[16] Francis Lange, interview with author, audiocassette, July 9, 2010.

[17] Gloria Yberra Sotello, interview by author, audiocassette, February 2013.

[18] Don Rivers, *Terrace Topics*, August 1942, 11.

[19] LuDean Harmsen Pontius, interview, videocassette, 1990. Also, telephone conversation with author, 2012.

[20] Norma Anderson, ed. , "Phyllis Burns," *San Memories*, 11.

[21] Victor Funk, interview, videocassette, 1990.

[22] Shih Hao Tsai, interview, videocassette, 1990.

[23] Mark Caldwell, *The Last Crusade: The War on Consumption*, 9.

[24] *Total Annual Cost of Operation and Income from Hennepin County Patients and Their Families. 1951*. Report prepared by the Hennepin County Tuberculosis Association. Unp.

[25] Ah-gwah-ching annual reports, folder 1961, 116.A.2.6, Minnesota Historical Society archives.

[26] *Minnesota's Health*, October 1961.

[27] "Treatment Practices, Outcomes, and Costs of Multidrug-Resistant and Extensively Drug-Resistant Tuberculosis, United States, 2005–2007," *Emerging Infectious Diseases*, Volume 20, Number 5—May 2014.

[28]Questions and answers about TB. <<http://www.cdc.gov/tb/publications/faqs/qa_TBDisease.htm#Active4.> Retrieved April 4, 2014.

[29]World Health Organization, Global Tuberculosis Report 2015. http://who/int/tb/publications/global_report?en/. Retrieved October 9, 2016.

[30]Tuberculosis, 2014. Minnesota Department of Health. <<www.health.state.mn/divs/idepc/newsletters/dcn/sum14/tb.html>> Retrieved October 9, 2016.

[31]Trends in Tuberculosis, 2014. National Center for HIV/AIDS, Viral Hepatitis, STC, and TB Prevention, Center for Disease Control. Retrieved October 8, 2016. <<http://www.cdc.gov/tb/publications/factsheets/statistics/tbtrends-2014.pdf >>

Bibliography

Annual reports. Ah-gwah-ching, Minnesota State Sanatorium, Walker, Minnesota. Accessed at Gale Family Library, Minnesota Historical Society.
———— Glen Lake Sanatorium, Oak Terrace, Minnesota. Accessed at Gale Family Library, Minnesota Historical Society.

Anderson, Norma. *San Memories: Glen Lake Sanatorium, Oak Terrace Nursing Home.* Self-published, 1990.

Bates, Barbara. *Bargaining for life: a social history of tuberculosis, 1876-1938.* Philadelphia: University of Pennsylvania Press, 1992.

Berliner, Emile. *Muddy Jim and Other Rhymes: 12 Illustrated Health Jingles for Children.* Washington, D.C., 1929. http://loc.gov. Retrieved July 17, 2013.

Bistodeau, Barbara Meyer. "The Cadet Nurse Corps." April 4, 2007. http://www.camdennews.org.

Black, Edwin. *Remarks relating to my spontaneous and unrehearsed testimony before the house judiciary committee's subcommittee on the constitution on the historical question of eugenics and racism.* Washington, D.C., December 6, 2011. http://judiciary.house.gov/hearings.pdf/black12062011.pdf. Retrieved October 6, 2012.

Bowker, Geoffrey C. & Susan L. Star. *Sorting Things Out: Classification and its consequences.* Cambridge: Massachusetts Institute of Technology Press, 1999.

Buikstra, Jane E. *Prehistoric Tuberculosis in the Americas.* Northwestern University Archeological Program, Scientific Papers, 1981.

Caldwell, Mark. *The Last Crusade: The War on Consumption, 1862-1954.* New York: Atheneum, 1988.

Carrington, Thomas Spees. *Tuberculosis Hospital and Sanatorium Construction.* New York: National Association for the Study and Prevention of Tuberculosis, 1911.

Collected studies. Glen Lake Sanatorium, Oak Terrace, Minnesota. Accessed at Gale Family Library, Minnesota Historical Society.

D'Antonio, Patricia, et al. *Nurses' Work: Issues across Time and Place.* New York: Springer Publishing Co., 2007.

Darity, William, Jr., ed., *Race, Radicalism, and Reform; selected papers, Abram L. Harris.* New Brunswick, New Jersey: Transaction Publishers, 1989.

Diamond, Jared. *Guns, Germs, and Steel.* New York: W. W. Norton & Co, 1997.

Diedrich, Lisa. *Treatments: Language, Politics, and the Culture of Illness.* Minneapolis: University of Minnesota Press, 2007.

Dormandy, Thomas L. *The White Death: A History of Tuberculosis.* New York: New York University Press, 1999.

Duffy, John. *The Sanitarians: A History of American Public Health.* Chicago: University of Illinois Press, 1990.

Emerson, Charles Phillips. *Essentials of Medicine, 13th edition.* Philadelphia: J.B. Lippincott Company, 1939.

Farmer, Paul. *Infections and Inequalities: The Modern Plagues.* Berkeley: University of California Press, 1999.

Fitzgerald, F. Scott. "Minnesota's Capital in the Role of Main Street," quoted in Matthew Joseph Broccoli, Judith Baughman, *F. Scott Fitzgerald on Authorship.* University of South Carolina Press, 1996.

Gale Family Library, Minnesota Historical Society. Newspaper collection.

——— Photograph collection.

Glen Lake subject files, 1916–1991. Glen Lake Sanatorium, Oak Terrace, Minnesota. Accessed at Gale Family Library, Minnesota Historical Society.

Glen Lake Sanatorium files, 1920–1962. Glen Lake Sanatorium, Oak Terrace, Minnesota. Accessed at Gale Family Library, Minnesota Historical Society.

Gohr, Glenn. "Got Any Rivers? The Story of an Inspirational Song." *Assemblies of God Heritage,* 16, no. 4, 1996–1997.

Grahn, Anya. Rise and Fall of the Tuberculosis Sanitarium [sic] in Response to the White Plague. Master of Science in Historic Preservation thesis. Ball State University, Muncie, IN, May 2012.

Hayes, Edward. *Tuberculosis As It Comes and Goes, 2nd edition.* Springfield, Illinois: Bannerstone House, 1947.

Hennepin County Medical Center. "Ambulance Service History." http://www.hcmc.org/education/ems/ems_dept/ambulance/history.htm. Retrieved June 21, 2010.

Hennepin County Review. Accessed at Hopkins Historical Society.

Hennepin County Tuberculosis Association. Reports. Accessed at Gale Family Library, Minnesota Historical Society.

Hennepin History Museum. Photograph collection.

Hippocrates. *Of the epidemics, Book I, Section 1, First Constitution.* Translated by Francis Adams. http://classics.mit.edu/Hippocrates/epidemics.1.i.html.

Holmes, Fred G. *Tuberculosis: A book for the patient.* New York: D. Appleton-Century Co., 1935.

Hopkins Historical Society. Photograph collection.

Hrubec, Zdenek and John D. Boice Jr., Richard R. Monson, et al. "Breast Cancer after Multiple Chest Fluoroscopies." *Cancer Research,* 49, 1989.

Husboe, Arthur R. and Nancy Owen Nelson. *Selected Letters of Frederick Manfred, 1932-1954.* Lincoln: University of Nebraska Press, 1988.

Kass, Amalie M. "A Brief History of the Channing Laboratory." http://www.channing.harvard.edu/kass.htm. Retrieved July 13, 2012.

Kathryn A. Martin Library, University of Minnesota–Duluth. Photograph collection.

Kawano, Martin. "Chapter 12: Glen Lake." Unpublished manuscript.

Krugerud, Mary. Interviews. Audiotape, phone calls, and video. Author's collection.

——— Personal correspondence. Emails and letters. Author's collection.

——— and Colleen Spadaccini. *From Beginning to End: Glen Lake Sanatorium and Oak Terrace Nursing Home.* Documentary, 1991.

Kurver, Harold. Interview by Thomas Saylor, March 18, 2002. http://www.lindavdahl.com/Bio%20Pages/H.Kurvers/H.Kurvers.bio.htm. Retrieved November 14, 2004.

Long, Esmond R. "Tuberculosis," *Preventive Medicine in World War II, Volume IV.* United States Army, Medical Department. http://history.amedd.army.mil/booksdocs/wwii/PM4/DEFAULT.htm. Retrieved April 7, 2014.

Maisel, Albert Q. "General Bradley Cleans up the Veterans' Hospitals." *Reader's Digest,* December 1945.

Maisel, Albert Q. "The Veteran betrayed," *Reader's Digest,* April 1945.

Maitland, Leslie. "The Design of Tuberculosis Sanatoria in Late Nineteenth Century Canada," *Bulletin of the Society for the Study of Architecture in Canada,* 14, no.1, 1989. http://dalspace.library.dal.ca/bitstream/handle/10222/71570/vol14_1_5_13.pdf?sequence=1. Retrieved April 4, 2014.

Mann, Thomas. *Magic Mountain*. Translated by John Woods. Everyman's Library, 2005.

"Maryanna Manfred papers." Accessed at Upper Midwest Literary Archives, University of Minnesota Libraries:

Mason, Jean S. "The Discourse of Disease: 'Patient Writes' at the 'University of Tuberculosis.'" http://web.english.ufl.edu/pnm/mason.html. Retrieved September 17, 2012.

Mattocks, Brewer. *Minnesota as a Home for Invalids*. Philadelphia: J.B. Lippincott Co., 1881.

Maxson, Gloria Stromseth. *Kennings*. Boston: Branden Press, 1974.

Mead, M. Nathaniel. "Benefits of Sunlight: A Bright Spot for Human Health," *Environmental Health Perspectives*, 116, 2008. http://www.ncbi.nlm.nih.gov/pmc/articles/PMC2290997. Retrieved June 15, 2014.

Medical staff/administrative meeting minutes, 1925–1988. Glen Lake Sanatorium, Oak Terrace, Minnesota. Accessed at Gale Family Library, Minnesota Historical Society.

Meyer, Roy W. *History of the Santee Sioux*. University of Nebraska Press, 1967.

Minneapolis city directories. Accessed at Gale Family Library, Minnesota Historical Society.

Minnesota History magazine. Accessed at Gale Family Library, Minnesota Historical Society.

"Minnesota State Fair History." http://www.mnstatefair.org/pdf/media/MSF_History.pdf. Retrieved August 2, 2016.

Miscellaneous minutes and reports, 1939–1991. Glen Lake Sanatorium, Oak Terrace, Minnesota. Accessed at Gale Family Library, Minnesota Historical Society.

Miscellaneous records, 1918–1991. Glen Lake Sanatorium, Oak Terrace, Minnesota. Accessed at Gale Family Library, Minnesota Historical Society.

National Tuberculosis Association. *A directory of sanatoria, hospitals and day camps for the treatment of tuberculosis in the United States*. 1919.

New York City. *Annual Report of the Board of Health of the Department of Health of the City of New York for the Year Ending December 31*. http://archive.org/details/annualreportsta00stagoog. Retrieved June 15, 2014.

Occupational therapy records, 1922–1935. Glen Lake Sanatorium, Oak Terrace, Minnesota. Accessed at Gale Family Library, Minnesota Historical Society.

Patient records and registers, 1916–1991. Glen Lake Sanatorium, Oak Terrace, Minnesota. Accessed at Gale Family Library, Minnesota Historical Society.

Pennsylvania Commonwealth. Department of Agriculture. *Tuberculosis of Cattle and the Pennsylvania Plan for Its Repression*, 75. http://www.archive.org/details/cu31924000379598. Retrieved March 5, 2012.

Pottenger, Francis M. *Tuberculosis and How to Combat It: A Book for the Patient*. St. Louis: C.V. Mosby Company, 1921.

Published records. Ah-gwah-ching, Minnesota State Sanatorium, Walker, Minnesota. Accessed at Gale Family Library, Minnesota Historical Society.

Reminisce magazine. Author's collection.

Rosenblatt, Milton. "Pulmonary tuberculosis: evolution of modern therapy." *Bulletin of the New York Academy of Medicine*, 49, no.3, March 1971.

Ross, William. *I Wanted to Live*. Wisconsin Tuberculosis Association, 1953.

Roth, Julius. *Timetables: Structuring the Passage of Time in Hospital Treatment and Other Careers*. New York: Bobbs-Merrill, 1963.

Ryan, Frank. *The Forgotten Plague: How the Battle against Tuberculosis was Won—and Lost*. Boston: Little, Brown and Company, 1993. First published as: *Tuberculosis: The Greatest Story Never Told*, England: Swift Publishers, 1992.

Sanborn, F.B., ed. *The Writings of Henry David Thoreau, VI, Familiar Letters*. Boston: Houghton Mifflin; Cambridge, Massachusetts: Riverside Press, 1906.

Seagrave, Sadie Fuller. *Saints' Rest*. St. Louis: C.V. Mosby, 1918.

Sherman, Irwin W. *Twelve diseases that changed our world*. Washington, D.C.: ASM Press, 2007.

Taylor, Robert. *Saranac: America's Magic Mountain*. New York: Paragon House Publishers, 1986.

Terrace Topics. 1933–1952. Accessed at Gale Family Library, Minnesota Historical Society.

Thomas, C.C. *With Their Dying Breath*. Corydon, Indiana: CCThomas Writing Solutions, 2007.

Trends in Tuberculosis, 2014. National Center for HIV/AIDS, Viral Hepatitis, STC, and TB Prevention, Center for Disease Control. http://www.cdc.gov/tb/publications/factsheets/statistics/tbtrends-2014.pdf. Retrieved October 8, 2016.

"Trudeau Elementary School." *Marshall University/High School Alumni Newsletter*, 19, no.1, 2011.

"Trudeau School of Tuberculosis—Historic Saranac Lake." http://localwi-ki.net/hsl/Trudeau_School_of_Tuberculosis. Retrieved September 21, 2013.

Tsuchida, John Hobuya. *Reflections: Memoirs of Japanese American Women in Minnesota,* Pacific Asia Press, 1995.

Tuberculosis Hospital and Sanatorium Directory. New York: National Tuberculosis Association, 1951.

Ulmer, Edgar. *Goodbye, Mr. Germ.* Film. National Tuberculosis Association, 1940.

United Nations Data. http://data.un.org.

Vavra, Helen Mary and Albert James Kranz. *The Dvoraks of Minnetonka Township, Minnesota.* Minneapolis: Albert Kranz, 1988.

Vocational training records, 1922–1935. Glen Lake Sanatorium, Oak Terrace, Minnesota. Accessed at Gale Family Library, Minnesota Historical Society.

Williams, David Eugene. "I Remember . . . Patsy's Cure." http://www.archive.thoracic.org/sections/about-ats/centennial/vignettes/articles/vignette4.html. Retrieved February 24, 2014.

World Health Organization. *Global Tuberculosis Report 2015.* http://who/int/tb/publications/global_report?en/. Retrieved October 9, 2016.

——— *Tuberculosis.* Fact sheet. October 2012.

Yamshchikov, Alexandra V, et al. "Vitamin D status and antimicrobial peptide cathelicidin (LL-37) concentrations in patients with active pulmonary tuberculosis." *American Journal of Clinical Nutrition,* 92, no. 3., September 2010.

Index